S0-BAZ-805

Livonia Public Library
ALFRED NOBLE BRANCH
32901 PLYMOUTH ROAD
Livonia, Michigan 48150-1793
(734)421-6600
LIVN #19

J616.4
G

I HAVE DIABETES.

NOW WHAT?

LESLIE C. GREEN

AND

PAT KELLY

Livonia Public Library
ALFRED NOBLE BRANCH
32901 PLYMOUTH ROAD
Livonia, Michigan 48150-1793
(734)421-6600
LIVN #19

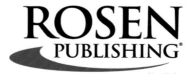

ROSEN
PUBLISHING®

New York

JAN 2 1 2013

Published in 2012 by The Rosen Publishing Group, Inc.
29 East 21st Street, New York, NY 10010

Copyright © 2012 by The Rosen Publishing Group, Inc.

First Edition

All rights reserved. No part of this book may be reproduced in any form without permission in writing from the publisher, except by a reviewer.

Library of Congress Cataloging-in-Publication Data

Green, Leslie.
I have diabetes. Now what? / Leslie Green, Pat Kelly. — 1st ed.
   p. cm. — (Teen life 411)
Includes bibliographical references and index.
ISBN 978-1-4488-4653-5 (library binding)
I. Kelly, Pat. II. Title.
RC660.4.G734 2012
616.4'62—dc22

                          2010045918

Manufactured in the United States of America

CPSIA Compliance Information: Batch #S11YA: For further information, contact Rosen Publishing, New York, New York, at 1-800-237-9932.

3 9082 12207 0413

CONTENTS

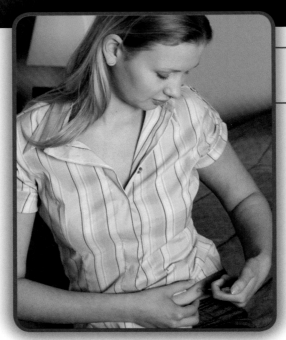

Diabetes affects around twenty-three million people in the United States and millions more worldwide. But what is it? Diabetes, technically known as diabetes mellitus, is a metabolic disorder that results from an imbalance of hormones produced in the pancreas. People with diabetes aren't able to properly convert the food they eat into nutrients needed by the body to function. This can be dangerous because without nutrients, the body is unable to function properly.

It is not contagious, meaning that it cannot spread from person to person. No one can catch diabetes from a person who has it. Diabetes is called a syndrome, which is a collection of diseases. This means that more than one type of diabetes exists. Diabetes is also something that often goes undiagnosed for a long time. The condition has a long incubation period, which is why

Performing injections on yourself can be scary at first, but once you do it a few times, it gets easier.

many children with diabetes are not diagnosed until puberty.

Having diabetes does not mean that a person will not be able to live a full and productive life. Having diabetes will not affect any goals or dreams. Many people who have diabetes are able to live happy and healthy lives. Actress Halle Berry, pop star Nick Jonas, professional football player Jay Cutler, and pro snowboarder Sean Busby are just some of the people who didn't let diabetes stop them from achieving their dreams.

WHAT ARE THE CAUSES OF DIABETES?

The body's immune system plays an important role in the development of diabetes. When functioning properly, the immune system protects the body from foreign substances, such as viruses and bacteria, which may enter it. For some reason that scientists have yet to fully understand, the immune system of a person with diabetes seeks out the cells that produce insulin and destroys them. This causes the body to stop producing insulin either partially or completely. Without the presence of insulin in the body, diabetes develops. Scientists are still trying to determine exactly what causes the immune system to attack these cells.

Heredity also plays a role in determining who will develop diabetes, especially type 2 diabetes. A person is at a higher risk for developing diabetes if someone in his or her family has or had diabetes.

THE PANCREAS

The pancreas is a long, thin organ that rests behind the stomach, next to the upper intestine. The pancreas is made up of two different kinds of tissue: exocrine and endocrine. The exocrine tissues make up the main part of the pancreas and produce enzymes used in digestion. The endocrine cells, about a million of them, are scattered in clumps throughout the entire pancreas. These are called the islets of Langerhans. These islets are made of three different types of cells, each producing or secreting a different hormone used in the body. The alpha cells secrete glucagon, the beta cells produce the protein insulin, and the delta cells produce the hormone somatostatin.

The first two, glucagon and insulin, are responsible for breaking down the food that enters the stomach, turning it into fuel that can be used by the body, and distributing it to the various parts of the body that need the fuel. The insulin-producing cells make up most of the islets. Glucagon works by increasing blood glucose levels while insulin works to decrease the blood glucose levels. Glucose that is in the blood is called blood sugar. When the alpha and beta cells work together properly, the body maintains a healthy amount of glucose, which is the main energy provider for the majority of bodily functions. Most of the food people eat is converted into the simple sugar glucose. Glucose is not the same as the sugar found in food. When people talk about sugar in relation to diabetes, they really mean glucose. The glucose level in the blood fluctuates in response to a person's daily activities, from eating a meal to exercising to entering stressful situations.

When the level of glucose in the body rises, for instance, after a person eats a meal, the body signals the pancreas to produce insulin. Insulin then signals muscle and fat tissue to absorb the amount of glucose needed for daily activities. Glucose that is not needed in the body at that time is stored in the liver in the form of a starch called glycogen. The body can access this reservoir of fuel whenever it is needed.

After a person exercises, the body usually needs more fuel, so the alpha cells then become more active, producing glucagon. Glucagon breaks down the glycogen and causes it to be released into the bloodstream for the body to use. This raises the level of blood sugar. In healthy people, the level always falls into set parameters (values).

In a person without diabetes, the amount of insulin and glucagon produced is balanced. If, however, the glucose level increases and the body is unable to use the extra sugar because the level of insulin is insufficient or because the body cannot absorb the insulin, then diabetes develops. Without enough insulin, cells cannot use the glucose in the blood and it builds up. The excess glucose cannot be stored in the liver and muscles, and when the glucose in the blood reaches a certain level, the body will force it out as waste, increasing urination.

DIABETES THROUGH TIME

Diabetes was first described in Egyptian writings around 1500 BCE. About 230 CE, a Greek physician named Aretaeus is believed to have called the disease "diabetes," which in Greek means "to siphon" or "to suck out." One of the symptoms of diabetes is excessive urination. He described diabetes as "the melting down of the flesh and limbs into urine." The word "diabetes" was used to describe how water seemed to pass right through the body of a person with the disease. Aretaeus wrote that a person with diabetes had an all-consuming thirst that resulted in constant urination. He thought that when a person with diabetes urinated, parts of the body were also swept away. He believed that the stomach lining, called the peritoneum, was the source of diabetes and so believed satisfying the stomach was the way to quench the patient's thirst. He suggested a diet that included a variety of remedies, such as drinking water mixed with apples and eating mixtures of dates, quince, and other fruits. Drinking milk mixed with groats or other cereal grains was the mainstay of the diet.

The urine of a person with diabetes contains a lot of extra sugar because the body is unable to break it down effectively. The word "mellitus," which is Latin for "honey," was added in 1679 to the term "diabetes" when a doctor tasted the urine of a person diagnosed with diabetes and said it was as sweet as honey.

Although diabetes had been around a long time, it wasn't until the mid-1800s that medical science began to understand more accurately what diabetes was and began to develop ways to treat it. Until the twentieth century if a person had diabetes, he or she usually died from it. Today, doctors understand even more about what diabetes is and how to help those with the

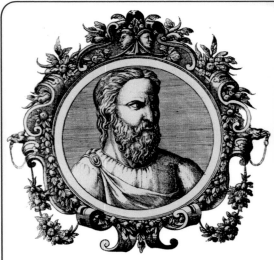

Aretaeus of Cappadocia, a Greek physician, is believed to be the first doctor to use the term "diabetes." One of the great doctors in history, Aretaeus is also credited with discovering celiac disease.

condition live normal and healthy lives. Nevertheless, doctors still don't know what exactly causes diabetes, and there is no cure for it yet.

Treatments for diabetes have varied greatly throughout the centuries, from drinking fruit wines to horseback riding, taking lukewarm baths to bloodletting to, eventually, using insulin.

THE INTRODUCTION OF INSULIN

In 1889, Dr. Joseph von Mering and Dr. Oskar Minkowski, who believed that there was a direct relationship between the pancreas and diabetes, began experimenting with dogs. They removed the pancreas from a healthy dog. The dog did not die immediately but began to urinate a lot, which is a symptom of diabetes. The doctors knew that the urine was sweet because the urine puddles attracted flies. Eventually, the dog went into a coma and died. The link between the pancreas and diabetes was established, and the search began to determine what in the pancreas caused diabetes.

About the same time, Paul Langerhans, a German medical student, was studying the pancreas. He grew curious about some cells that looked different from most of the other cells in the organ. These cells were later named the islets of Langerhans. Other scientists experimented with these cells and determined that if they were removed from the pancreas, diabetes developed.

In 1910, Dr. Edward Sharpey-Schafer of Scotland decided that a chemical he called insulin was missing from the pancreas of people with diabetes.

In 1921, at the University of Toronto, doctors Frederick Banting and Charles Best continued the experiments of Mering and Minkowski but carried them one step further. The scientists believed that insulin was manufactured in the pancreas in the islets of Langerhans. To investigate this idea, they first removed the pancreas from healthy dogs, causing them to

Charles Best (left) and Frederick Banting (right) are shown here with one of their test subjects. Their experiments, which led to the discovery of insulin, changed diabetes from a death sentence to an illness that could be controlled.

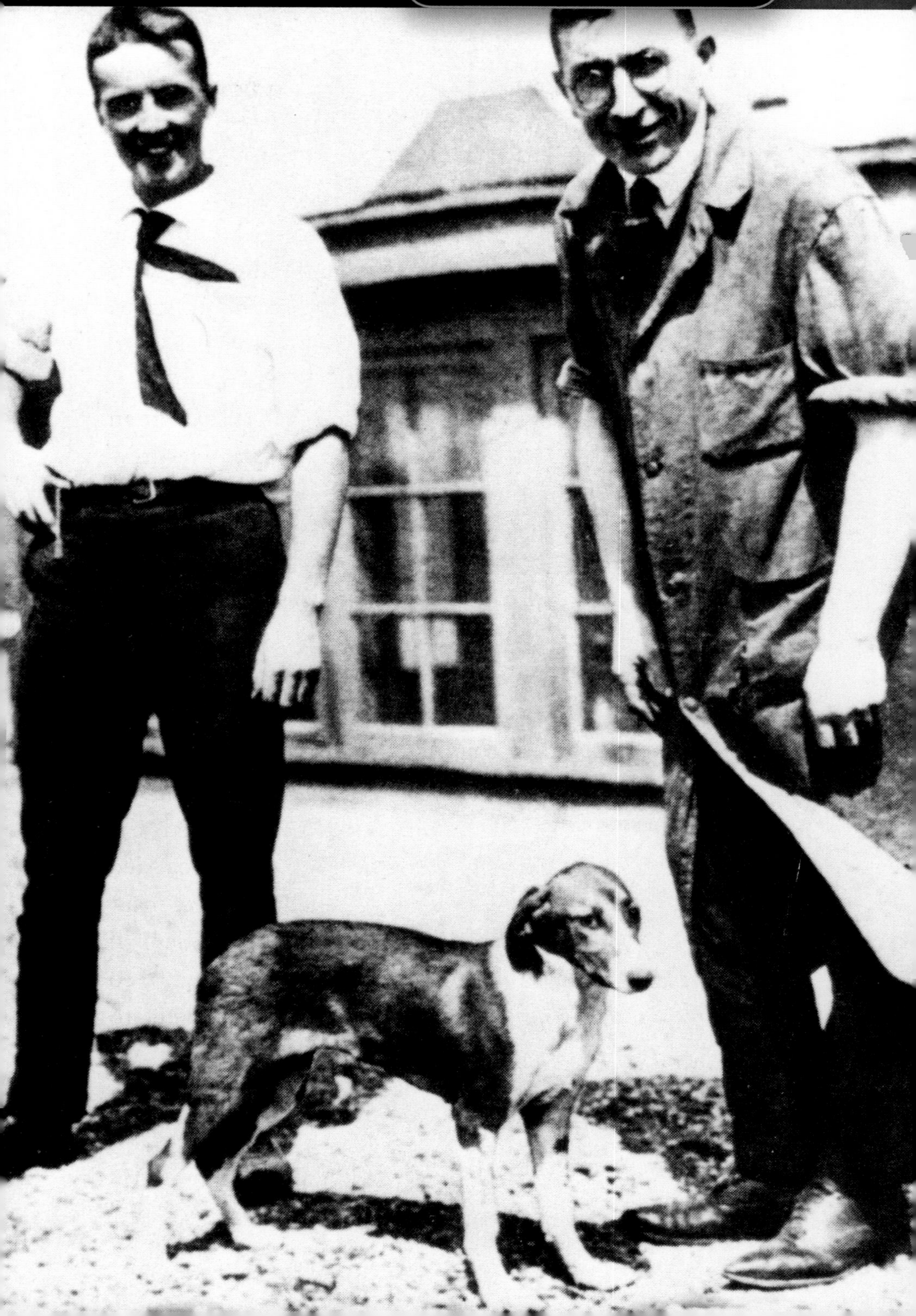

develop diabetes. They then took fluid from the islets of Langerhans in healthy dogs—those that still had their pancreas—and injected it into the sick dogs. The effect on the sick dogs was dramatic: it stopped their symptoms.

Banting and Best then teamed up with J. B. Collip to extract a more refined form of insulin from cattle. With the help of a team of researchers under the direction of Dr. J. J. R. Macleod, these four men developed insulin as a treatment for diabetes. That same year, an oral dose of insulin was tested on Dr. Joe Gilchrist. Nothing seemed to happen. Early the next year, Leonard Thompson, a patient in Toronto Hospital, was injected with insulin on two different occasions and his condition improved. In May of 1922, Macleod officially announced the discovery of insulin. Finally, people with diabetes were given some hope. Insulin is still the key to controlling diabetes. It is not a cure but a treatment that makes diabetes easier to live with.

Until the 1980s, the only type of insulin available for people with diabetes came from the pancreases of animals, mostly cows and hogs. Today, there is a variety of insulin available: cow, hog, cow-hog combinations, and, most common, human insulin. Human insulin is made from a combination of hog insulin (because it is closest to human insulin) and genetic engineering. Human insulin is quickly becoming the most popular insulin because of its purity and its fast absorption into the bloodstream.

Different Types of Diabetes

Diabetes is divided into two main types: insulin dependent and non-insulin dependent.

Type 1 Diabetes

Type 1 diabetes, also known as insulin-dependent diabetes or insulin-dependent diabetes mellitus (IDDM), used to be called juvenile-onset diabetes because it seemed to appear only during childhood or adolescence. Now doctors know that it can appear at any time in life.

Type 1 diabetes is an autoimmune disorder that stems from the destruction of the insulin-producing cells in the pancreas. The body produces little or no insulin and is unable to lower the level of glucose. Glucose accumulates in the blood, raising a person's blood sugar level. This is called hyperglycemia or high blood sugar. When the blood sugar level gets too high, glucose is removed from the body in urine as waste. As a result, someone with high blood sugar may have to go to the bathroom as often as his or her body needs to get rid of extra glucose. Frequent urination can result in a substantial loss of water, because water is a main component of urine. This water loss, known as dehydration, can lead to great thirst, dry mouth, blurry vision, and dry skin.

Also, if cells cannot get the glucose they need, they "starve." This may make a diabetic person feel very hungry even when he or she has just finished eating. If someone has diabetes, his or her body does not produce the fuel it needs and that person may often feel weak and tired. Weight loss may also occur as the body's demands for fuel force fat cells to break down. In addition, high glucose levels can damage nerves, which may result in a tingling feeling in the feet or leg cramps at night. High glucose levels also interfere with the action of white blood cells, which can slow the healing of cuts. High glucose levels make it easier for bacteria to grow and may result in a variety of skin infections.

If hyperglycemia is not treated, the result can be diabetic ketoacidosis (DKA) coma. When there is not enough insulin, the body looks for alternative fuel. That alternative fuel is fat. When fat is broken down into energy, it produces a poisonous waste called ketone. Ketones accumulate in the blood and eventually in the urine. If the condition is not treated, the person will lose consciousness and possibly die.

Insulin-dependent diabetes affects males and females equally. Treatment for type 1 diabetes includes daily injections of insulin to help the body use the glucose it needs. Insulin treatment is often balanced with diet and exercise.

Type 2 Diabetes

Type 2 diabetes, also called insulin-resistant or non-insulin-dependent diabetes mellitus (NIDDM), used to be called adult-onset diabetes because it normally occurs in adults over the age of forty. But as with type 1 diabetes, doctors realized that type 2 diabetes could appear at

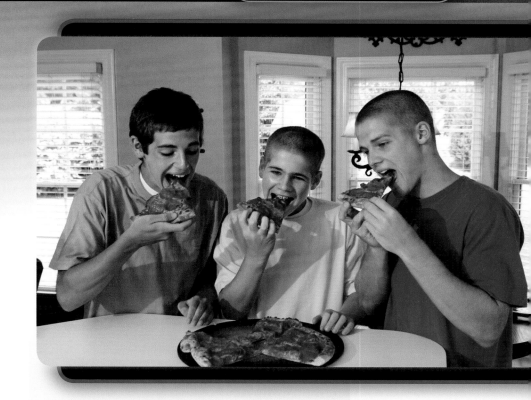

A person who is diagnosed with diabetes must learn how to control his or her eating habits. A little pizza once in a while is OK, but be sure to monitor your blood sugar.

any age. Type 2 diabetes often, but not always, strikes those who are overweight or obese.

In Type 2 diabetes, the body doesn't produce enough insulin, or it produces enough insulin but doesn't use it properly or resists it. When type 2 diabetes is diagnosed in young people, it is called maturity onset diabetes in the young, or MODY. Type 2 diabetes affects mostly

GESTATIONAL DIABETES

Gestational diabetes occurs only in pregnant women. About 4 percent of all pregnant women develop this form of diabetes, and most of them have no prior history of any type of diabetes. (If a woman has been diagnosed with diabetes before becoming pregnant, she has pre-gestational diabetes.) So far no one knows for certain what causes gestational diabetes, but scientists have some ideas.

Hormones from the placenta that help the baby grow also inhibit the mother's ability to absorb glucose. This causes insulin resistance, which can lead to high levels of glucose in the blood (hyperglycemia). The treatment for gestational diabetes is a combination of careful diet, exercise, and sometimes insulin injections. The American Diabetes Association (ADA) believes that all women should be tested for gestational diabetes in their sixth month of pregnancy, which is when insulin requirements for the mother increase.

After a mother with gestational diabetes gives birth, her insulin resistance usually disappears. Women who have had gestational diabetes frequently develop it again during subsequent pregnancies. Many of them also develop type 2 diabetes later in life. Proper diet and exercise are important tools in a healthy lifestyle and will help prevent or delay the onset of type 2 diabetes and its many complications.

females but can affect males as well. You are at higher risk for developing type 2 diabetes if someone in your family has it or if you are overweight or obese.

Setting up a healthy diet and exercise plan for the patient is the usual treatment for this type of diabetes. For overweight people with type 2 diabetes, weight loss often helps the body use the insulin better. Some people with type 2 diabetes are also treated with insulin.

Millions of people have type 2 diabetes, and health care professionals are alarmed at the increasing number of young people who develop this disease. In today's world, junk food, fast food, sodas, and foods high in calories seem to be part of the everyday diet of many young people, at home and in school. Many of the newly diagnosed diabetics also suffer from obesity.

Brittle Diabetes

Brittle diabetes, also called unstable diabetes or labile diabetes, occurs when a person's blood sugar level goes from one extreme to another for no apparent reason. This rising and falling cannot be predicted and may not be preceded by any symptoms. Sometimes, people confuse brittle diabetes with type 1 diabetes. Another common misconception is that all teens with diabetes have brittle diabetes. People assume this because blood glucose levels often fluctuate during puberty. These fluctuations, however, are not the same as those that characterize brittle diabetes. The blood sugar of people with brittle diabetes is frequently out of control.

CHAPTER 2

Many people are unaware of the symptoms of diabetes. It's important to recognize these symptoms, especially if someone in your family has any type of diabetes or if you have had these symptoms for more than a short time. If you or someone you know experiences any of these symptoms, seek medical attention immediately. Many people who have diabetes, especially type 2 diabetes, are unaware that they have the disease. If it is not treated properly, diabetes can be fatal. The sooner you find out, the sooner you can treat the condition.

Also remember that just because you have one or more of these symptoms, it doesn't mean you have diabetes. And not everyone who has diabetes has all, or even some, of these symptoms. The only way to be sure is to be tested for diabetes by a doctor. If you have these symptoms, talk to your parents and let them know what's going on so that they can follow up with an appointment with your doctor.

The following list describes the general symptoms that many people with diabetes experience:

- Frequent urination (polyuria)
- Continual thirst or dry mouth (polydipsia)
- Always feeling hungry (polyphagia)
- Tiredness and weakness

- Weight loss
- Blurry vision
- Numbness or tingling in feet or legs
- Skin infections or slow-to-heal cuts
- Extremely dry skin

TESTING FOR DIABETES

When you visit your doctor, you may be asked to have a screening test. A screening test requires a drop of blood and can tell your doctor if you might have diabetes. If this test indicates that diabetes is likely, the doctor will then perform a diagnostic test that will determine for certain whether you have diabetes. You should be in relatively good health when you have these tests done. A cold or other kind of illness can cause a problem getting the correct readings. The following sections discuss some of the tests your doctor might perform.

Fasting Plasma Glucose Test

For this test, you don't eat or drink anything overnight, usually for about eight hours. Then the doctor takes a sample of your blood for analysis. Plasma is the part of your blood that carries solid cells, which would include glucose. So this is a test for blood sugar. Normal fasting plasma glucose levels are less than 126 mg/dl. Mg/dl stands for milligrams per deciliter. A deciliter is 1/10 of a liter. A milligram is 1/1000 of a gram. (A paper clip weighs a gram.) For every deciliter of blood, normal fasting glucose levels should show less than 126

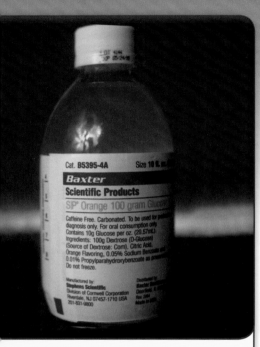

Sometimes called glucola, this glucose beverage is used in diagnosing diabetes using the glucose tolerance test. Some doctors have started using jelly beans instead, since they produce the same result.

milligrams. If the test is higher than that, the doctor will do the test again.

In the past, if two or more tests showed a glucose level greater than 140 mg/dl, the doctor would diagnose you with diabetes. With the new American Diabetes Association guidelines, doctors consider fasting plasma glucose levels above 126 milligrams to indicate the possibility of diabetes. A person who has a fasting plasma glucose level of 126 mg/dl is considered to have an impaired ability to process glucose. A person whose fasting plasma glucose level is 140 mg/dl or more is considered to have provisional diabetes until another test on another day confirms the same results. If the results on both days are the same, the person will be diagnosed as having diabetes.

Oral Glucose Tolerance Test

Although the ADA has decided that the fasting plasma glucose tolerance test is sufficient to diagnose diabetes, some doctors may recommend the oral glucose tolerance test. Ask if this test is absolutely necessary because it can be very expensive and unpleasant.

You must fast overnight before this test as well. In the morning, the doctor takes a blood sample. Then you drink about seventy-five grams of glucose, and your blood is tested at intervals, five times during three hours, to measure your glucose levels. A person without diabetes will show a quick rise and fall in glucose levels after each drink. This is a result of the infusion of glucose and then the insulin response. A person with diabetes will show a rise that does not come down very quickly, indicating insufficient or lack of insulin. The oral glucose tolerance test does not determine whether you have diabetes, but it does indicate impaired glucose tolerance. If your doctor suspects diabetes, he or she will order additional tests before a diagnosis can be made.

Insulin C-Peptide Test

This is another blood test done after overnight fasting. The C-peptide test is given to determine how much insulin a person produces. In a person with type 1 diabetes, these peptide levels will measure zero, which indicates no insulin. In a person with type 2 diabetes, the peptide range will be normal or above normal, which indicates plenty of or too much insulin.

Islet-Cell Antibody Test

Scientists have developed an antibody test that predicts if a person will eventually develop diabetes. This test is

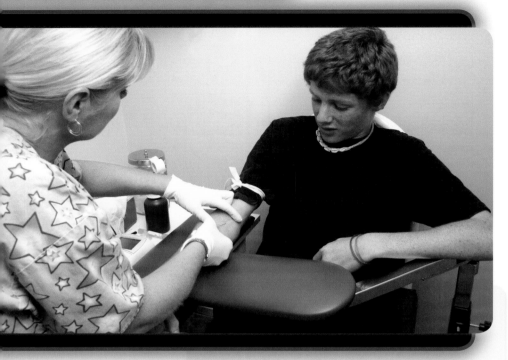

A nurse draws blood from a patient during an insulin C-peptide test. The blood sample is checked to see how much insulin (if any) the body produces after a fast.

often given to those who have family members with diabetes and want to know if they will develop the disease as well. Because diabetes develops over a long period of time, researchers are able to identify, before diabetes develops, people who may get the disease. The islet-cell antibody test is used to detect the presence of this particular antibody in a person's bloodstream. Not every family member feels the need to know ahead of time if he or she is going to develop a disease. If someone does want to know, however, this test is available.

CHAPTER 3

Although some people are more likely to get diabetes than others, diabetes can affect anyone at any time. About 23.6 million people in the United States, or 7.8 percent of the population, have diabetes. Of these 23.6 million, only 17.9 million have actually been diagnosed, whereas the other 5.7 million have no idea that they have the disease. Consider these interesting statistics:

- Each year, 1.6 million new cases of diabetes in people ages 20 or over are diagnosed.
- Between 5 and 10 percent of all cases of diabetes are type 1.
- About 90 to 95 percent of all cases of diabetes are type 2.
- Nine out of ten diabetic Americans have type 2 diabetes.

Type 1 diabetes is the kind of diabetes that you would find in most young people who have diabetes. This kind is also called insulin-dependent diabetes (because people who have it need to give themselves insulin shots to stay healthy). It is also called juvenile diabetes or juvenile-onset diabetes because it usually starts in childhood.

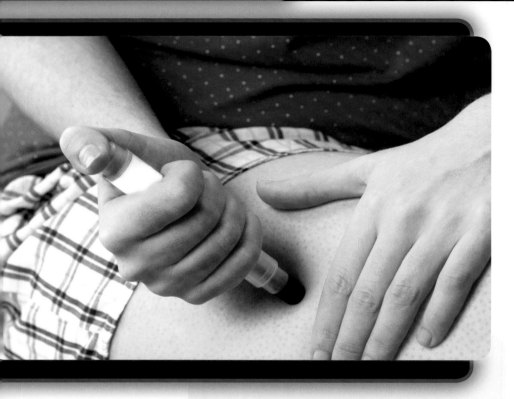

A girl with diabetes administers an injection of insulin using a pen injector. Pen injectors make it faster and easier to get the necessary insulin into the body.

Type 2 diabetes usually appears in people who are forty years old or older, have a family history of diabetes, are overweight and do not exercise regularly, and are of certain racial and ethnic groups (most commonly African American, Hispanic American, Asian and Pacific Islander, and Native American). It also appears in women who have had gestational diabetes.

Type 2 diabetes is currently on the rise because the number of older people in America is steadily increasing, and many of these older people are overweight and do not get enough exercise. Other types of diabetes include gestational diabetes, which only affects pregnant women (about 4 percent of them), and diabetes caused by such factors as another chronic illness, genetic syndromes, malnutrition, drugs, and surgery.

GENETICS AND DIABETES

Although having someone with diabetes in your family increases your chances of developing diabetes yourself, it does not mean that you will definitely get it. If you have a sibling or a parent with type 1 diabetes, your chance of developing it is about 10 to 25 percent because you may have inherited a family tendency toward diabetes. Of course, if your identical twin has diabetes, your chance of developing it increases to between 25 and 50 percent.

DIABETES AND RACE

As mentioned before, anyone can get diabetes. People all over the world are diagnosed with diabetes every day. If you think you are alone with your diabetes, here's a breakdown for you to consider. This is a sampling of people in various populations and the number of cases of diabetes:

- African Americans: approximately 11.8 percent and growing
- Mexican Americans: approximately 11.9 percent and growing
- Native Americans: 14.2 percent; in some tribes, 50 percent of the population has diabetes and this number is growing
- Puerto Ricans: approximately 12.6 percent
- Cuban Americans: approximately 8.2 percent

Of course, this is just a sampling of the people in the United States who get diabetes. Diabetes occurs all over the world. The United States is somewhere in the middle range. The point is that diabetes is everywhere. You are certainly not alone!

YOU HAVE DIABETES... NOW WHAT?

When someone is first diagnosed with diabetes, he or she will probably experience a wide range of emotions: denial, anger, guilt, depression, grief, and fear. You may feel all, some, or even none of these emotions. None of these reactions are wrong. All of them are perfectly normal. These feelings can come in any order and return from time to time. They become a problem only when they are not followed by acceptance and the desire to cope with diabetes.

Denial

Denial is a common reaction. "Well, the doctors must be wrong. I couldn't possibly have diabetes. I just won't think about it." Although denial is a natural reaction, it is also dangerous if it goes on too long. Diabetes is generally not diagnosed until people are in their early teens, after they have had it for some time. It is important to find a way to accept that you have diabetes so that you can move forward and begin to take control of it. That way you can live a long and productive life, as do many people with diabetes.

Anger and Guilt

It is OK to be angry. It's natural for a person who hears bad news to say it isn't fair or ask, "Why me?" Some teens feel guilty because they get diabetes. They think if they hadn't eaten all that junk food or if they had eaten more fruit, they wouldn't have diabetes. The truth is that there is no single cause of diabetes, and no one deserves to be sick. Diseases are not punishments. Often they are the result of many factors, some of which are beyond our control. No one wants to have diabetes, but it is something that just happens sometimes.

Grief, Fear, and Depression

Depression is another common response to being diagnosed with a disease. When you first learn that you have diabetes, you may feel very sad, almost as if you've lost

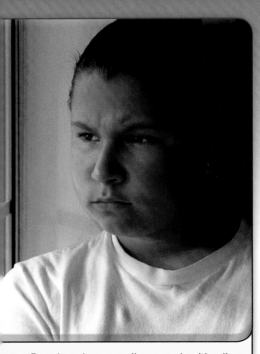

People who are diagnosed with diabetes can experience a variety of emotions, from denial to anger. During the time after your diagnosis, it's important to surround yourself with caring friends and family members.

someone important to you. In a way you have, and it's OK to grieve for that loss of the perfect self you thought you had. Yesterday everything was fine, and today you have a chronic disease. But, as with denial, depression that lasts too long can adversely affect your ability to deal properly with diabetes and could have long-term harmful effects. You may want to try keeping a diary about your feelings. Expressing your feelings, whether in writing, in person, by phone, or through e-mail to a parent, another relative, or a close friend, might make it easier for you to cope with those emotions as they occur.

It is understandable that a person can get tired of having to do all the things that are required to control diabetes. There are so many things a person would rather do than monitor blood glucose every day, eat a healthy diet, and exercise. But right now there is no cure, and until there is one, no one can decide not to be a diabetic anymore. If you do not try to control your diabetes now, you increase the risk of many diabetes-related complications and early death. There is no easy way around diabetes. It is up to you to keep your diabetes under control to ensure that you have a healthy future. If you feel like you just want to give up, try talking to a friend or counselor. Be open about how you feel. There is nothing wrong with feeling like giving up from time to time. The problem begins when you act on those feelings. By sharing these emotions with someone else, you can get a better sense of what you need to do.

ART'S STORY

My mom sacrificed her life to give me life. She was diagnosed with type 1 diabetes in 1971, when she was sixteen years old. Type 1 diabetes was a new disease that doctors knew very little about. Later on, my mother was given a suggestion not to have a child because it could endanger her life, and mine, too. She decided to ignore all of these suggestions just so I could experience the joy of life.

To this very day my mom still struggles with diabetes. She always has to test her blood sugar before she eats to make sure that she won't have a reaction. If her blood sugar is very low, she has to eat something sugary like orange juice, soda, or ice cream. If her blood sugar is too high, she has to take a shot of insulin.

There have been many times that my mom has gone into a very serious and dangerous diabetic reaction. One time we were staying at a friend's house, and I woke up and went to check on my mom. I found her sopping wet and moaning and screaming in bed. I was so frightened. I immediately called an ambulance and I couldn't remember the address that I was staying at. My mind focused on my mom and my mom only. It took the ambulance almost two and a half minutes to arrive. To me it felt like ten, and ten of the most miserable, surreal, longest minutes of my entire life. When the ambulance finally arrived, they gave her an IV, and in three minutes she was waking up slowly but surely.

There have been other times where I have had to take the initiative and help my mom out. The older I get the more time I spend away from my house and my mom. As I am nearing my final lap in my high school race, I feel that I need to slow down or go back to take care of my mom. I was given some advice from my mom's uncle who told me that it wasn't my responsibility to take care of her. I thought about whether my mom gave birth to me so I could stay and take care of her. She gave birth to me so I could experience life. If someone close to you has diabetes, it isn't your responsibility to take care of him or her.

—Art

(To share your story, please see page 154.)

CHAPTER 4

Having diabetes will change many things about the way you live.

- First of all, diabetes is a chronic condition that needs to be monitored and treated daily. You will be responsible for monitoring your blood sugar levels, watching for ketones in your urine and keeping a log of all the results, and, of course, taking your insulin every day.

- Second, you will be responsible for watching your diet and exercise so that they are in balance with your insulin intake. You will be responsible for saying no when someone offers you something you know will affect your diabetes.

- Third, and perhaps the hardest part of having diabetes as a teenager, you will have to assume a great deal of responsibility for yourself. You probably are used to your parents taking care of you when you are sick. Your mother or father also decides when you go to the doctor and when you take medicine. Someone older than you is usually responsible for taking your temperature if you aren't feeling well. Teenagers must learn to take responsibility for their own health. Although you will have a lot of help from

YOUR NEW LIFE WITH DIABETES

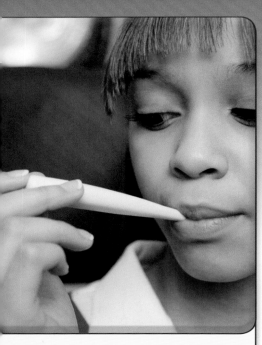

As you become an adult, you must learn how to take responsibility for your diabetes. Things like taking your own temperature and knowing when to call your doctor become important skills to learn.

your health care team, you will be the main caretaker. Your health care team will rely on you for a lot of the information they will need to help you control your diabetes. Many choices about diet and exercise will be made by you when you are not at home. You will have to take the time out to take care of your diabetes and yourself. If you don't, you run the risk of extremely serious health problems as you grow older. Remember that what you do today will affect the rest of your life. There is no room for risk taking with diabetes.

• Fourth, you will have to make time in your schedule for doctor visits. You should learn more about diabetes so that you know what your health care providers are talking about. Make them talk to you, not just to your parents. After all, you are the one with the disease.

ACCEPTANCE OF DIABETES

Having diabetes is not an easy thing, and it will require you to change your life, but it is something you must learn to accept even if it makes you angry at times. When you start to get upset, think about the following question: what part of having diabetes worries you the most?

- Daily testing and injections?
- Feeling different?
- Diet?
- Exercise?
- Getting sick?
- Dying?

Let's take these one at a time and see if we can come up with some solutions. If it's the daily testing and injections that are bothering you, you still have to ask why. Is it because they take so much time? Actually they take only a few minutes out of your day, so it can't be that.

Is it because the injections hurt? This may concern a lot of teens because many people do not like needles. Sometimes the injections may hurt, but there are some things you can do to relieve that, such as rubbing the injection site with a piece of ice before you put in the needle. Also, it helps to pinch a large section of the site when you inject the needle. If one site hurts, try another. You might also ask your doctor if there is a topical anesthetic on the market that you can use to numb the area. You should also think about how much better you feel once you have given yourself the insulin. If your injections continue to hurt, talk to your doctor or your diabetes educator. They may be able to suggest a different way to give yourself the injections so they do not hurt. You may want to try out different types of syringes to find the one that suits you best. Today's needles have a special coating that makes those injections less painful. If the injections really bother you that much, you may want to consider getting a pump. But remember, having a pump means that you accept responsibility for testing several times a day.

If you are worried about how you are going to test and take injections at school, talk this over with your parents and your teachers. If you can, plan your testing and injections between classes. If that isn't practical, you can either perform the procedures in class or leave class to go somewhere else, like to the school nurse's office. If you are going to test and inject insulin in class, be certain to tell your teacher ahead of time so that he or she won't be caught by surprise. Try testing in your lap. Chances are no one will even notice. But if they do, remember it is normal for your classmates to be curious at first. After a few times, this will all seem routine to them as well as to you, and no one will pay attention. If you prefer to test outside of the classroom, let your teacher know ahead of time that you will be leaving the class for a short time. Also you might want to research insulin pumps and see if pumping might be a good option for you.

Are you afraid that having diabetes makes you different somehow? Remember that millions of people have diabetes. There are 17.9 million people in the United States alone with diabetes. That is a lot of "different" people.

If your fear is really that people will look at you differently or treat you differently if they learn you have diabetes, it's possible that some people will. This can be especially difficult for teens. People you thought were your friends or schoolmates may not know anything about the disease, but they will make assumptions that may be hurtful. If someone makes hurtful assumptions or comments because you have diabetes, it shows that he or she lacks knowledge about the disease and, more important, it shows a lack of sincerity. If this happens, turn to friends who are honest and try to talk it out. True friends will stick with you no matter what. True friends will be concerned and will try to make you feel at ease. The teen years are often the most difficult years of anyone's life for different reasons. Some may feel left out or different because they can't afford fashionable clothes, or they wear glasses, or they just don't seem to be as popular as other people. This is also a time of shifting friendships for everyone, not just you. Try to remember that others are going through the same fear of rejection but for different reasons.

Are you afraid that you might not read the tests correctly or that you might give yourself the wrong amount of insulin? There are ways to prevent these things from happening. Practice reading the test strips before you give yourself an injection. Ask your diabetes educator to recommend test strips that he or she thinks would be good for you. Think about getting a glucose monitor that does the reading for you. If you are afraid that you are going to give yourself the wrong amount of insulin, remember that you and your health care provider have discussed dosages. You know how to match your glucose level and your insulin requirements with diet and exercise. If you still feel unsure, call your health care provider or get in touch with a diabetes educator who can walk you through it again.

What else can you do to make sure you are getting the right dosage? Make certain your syringe is calibrated to match your insulin vial. Be aware of the symptoms of high blood sugar (hyperglycemia) and low blood sugar (hypoglycemia). Do your self-monitoring of blood glucose (SMBG) at least four times a day. Learn to recognize when you need to adjust your dosage. Maintain a healthy balance between diet, exercise, and insulin. These things will come naturally to you over time. But if you've just been diagnosed, don't be afraid to call a member of your health care team for more information or reassurance. Get to know someone who has had diabetes for a while. Talk to that person and learn about his or her experiences. Ask lots of questions. There is no such thing as a stupid question. The more you know, the better you will be able to handle having diabetes.

Are you concerned that you will not like the diet or that you might eat the wrong foods? Dieting doesn't mean just eating lettuce and rice cakes. There is no longer any such thing as a "diabetic diet." A healthy diet includes everything you've already been eating, but in moderation. You can still have a piece of pie now and then, but you have to balance your insulin intake as well. Your health care team probably includes a dietitian who can help you plan healthy and delicious meals. Learn to read the nutrition information panel on food packaging. If you have type 2 diabetes, you must control your diet. Diet and exercise are the main methods for controlling blood sugar in type 2 diabetes. If you are worried about going out to eat or how to deal with eating at someone else's house, there are some things you can do. You will probably know ahead of time if you are going to a restaurant, so you can plan your insulin intake and exercise levels accordingly. Then as long as you don't go overboard, you'll have no problem. If going to a restaurant is a last-minute decision, you can order a salad or an appetizer and use that in place of one of your snacks. Ask for salad dressing or sauces on the side. Don't order fried foods. Remember to test your glucose levels as soon as you can. If you are invited to a friend's house and no one there knows you have diabetes, you will have time to plan for the meal. Eat small amounts. You don't have to eat everything that is put in front of you.

You may be worried about exercising, or you may just not want to exercise on certain days. Doctors recommend that exercise be part of everyone's life, not just people with diabetes. Exercise can make you feel and look well and will ensure a long and healthy life.

One of the best exercises you can do is walking. Not only will it help keep your weight under control, but walking as well as other exercises helps reduce stress by causing the body to release endorphins, the feel-good hormones. Again, just as with diet, you have to balance exercise and your insulin intake.

Are you worried about getting sick? Such feelings are normal, and that's why it's important to take precautions to avoid getting sick. If you are worried about common illnesses such as colds and the flu, talk to your doctor. He or she can give you some commonsense rules to reduce your chances of getting sick. Remember, you should have a flu shot every year. But if you do get sick and have to stay in bed, there are some general diabetes sick day rules that you can follow. The most important thing to remember is to take your insulin, drink a lot of fluids, and get plenty of rest. If you are worried about getting sick as a result of diabetes complications, remember that you can help delay or even prevent many of the complications by starting to take care of yourself and taking control of your diabetes now.

Are you worried about dying? Before the 1920s and the isolation of insulin, if you were diagnosed with diabetes you would die before the year was out. But the discovery of insulin has changed all that. People with diabetes live long, full, and productive lives if they take care of themselves.

Although it is normal to have worries about being a person with diabetes, too much worry can cause unnecessary stress. If you find you cannot stop worrying, you need to talk with your health care team about ways to minimize your worries. You may also want to talk to other people with diabetes to learn how they deal with their worries. Just as you can take control of your diabetes, you can take control of your worries.

STRESS

Everyone knows that stress is a part of everyday life. But too much stress from worry, anxiety, depression, anger, guilt, or even a physical ailment can increase blood sugar levels and lead to hyperglycemia. Stress releases additional hormones into the bloodstream that work to raise the blood sugar level. Stress can also lead to deeper depression. A person may not always be able to get rid of a source of stress. Sometimes a person can't even say why he or she feels stressed.

You need to learn how to cope with stress and combat it. When you feel stressed, try to find the cause. If you can identify the sources of stress, then you can begin to deal with them. Of course you can't take care of everything at once, but you can start small and work your way up. Counseling is a very good way to get help in identifying sources of stress. While the source of stress may not be your having diabetes, remember that stress itself can affect your health.

We tend to have some very recognizable physiological reactions to stress. We clench our teeth or jaws. We breathe quickly and shallowly. We tighten our neck muscles and hunch up our shoulders. We clench our fists, grind our teeth, and sweat. We feel our hearts beat faster. Learn to recognize these stress symptoms and work to reverse them.

Using deep breathing as an initial response to stress can help reduce its immediate effects. Gradually tighten and release all of your muscles several times. Take a moment away from the situation to decompress.

Exercise is very helpful because it releases endorphins. And exercise will help you keep in shape. That will also add to your positive self-image. Meditation exercises work, too. Find a quiet place to sit. Practice some deep breathing. Then think only of pleasant things. If a thought you don't like crosses your mind, quickly think of something else. Meditation may seem difficult at first, but it will get easier each time you do it.

HOW WILL DIABETES AFFECT MY FAMILY?

When you were first diagnosed, probably everyone in your family was confused about what having diabetes meant and how it would affect the family. A diagnosis of diabetes does change family dynamics and requires everyone to develop different coping skills. First, family members must learn to integrate diabetes into their daily lives. The first step toward this is learning as much as possible about the disease. Your doctor and other health care professionals can give you and your family a lot of information. There are also other resources, such as the ADA and the Juvenile Diabetes Foundation (JDF). You and other family members may want to join a diabetes support group. The ADA has an office in every state that has a list of educational services and support groups.

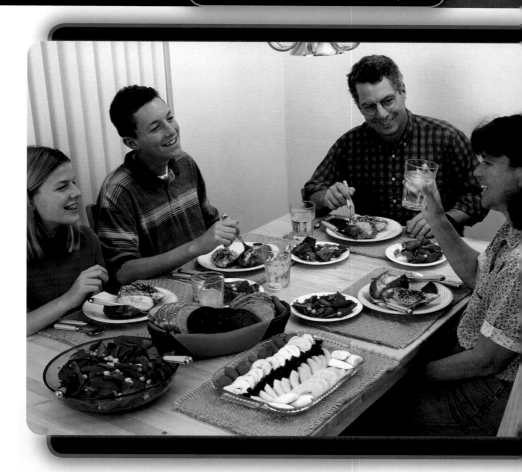

Part of learning how to control your diabetes means making some changes to your diet. But you don't have to do it alone. Talk to your parents about how you can learn how to cook healthier meals as a family.

If your diabetes requires insulin injections, both you and your parents have to learn how to do this. It can be scary at first, but usually you are allowed to practice on oranges or something similar. No one is sent home from the hospital with a syringe and some insulin and no training. Remember, you are not injecting anything into a vein, so relax. Everyone in the family should be taught the warning signs of hypoglycemia and hyper-glycemia and should know what to do in an emergency.

Chances are the family diet may have to be changed to accommodate diabetes. The good news is that this diet is probably healthier for everyone. It is a good idea for your family to stop buying junk food for a while until you are in control of your diabetes. That way you won't be tempted and won't feel resentful about what other family members are eating. You and your parents will have to learn how to share information with each other and how to ask necessary questions when you go to the doctor.

Second, but even more important, you and your family are going to have to come to terms with one another about wants and expectations concerning your diabetes. You cannot expect that your parents will immediately let you resume life as usual, and your parents can't expect that you will become a different person all of a sudden. You and your family may have to learn how to man-age stress more effectively because having a child with a chronic disease such as diabetes or being the person with diabetes can increase the stress within a family, especially in the beginning. The family will have to learn how to adapt. A counselor may be needed and is almost always helpful in teaching family members new ways of coping. Diabetes support groups are another resource for family members to talk about their problems and learn how other people in similar situations have handled them.

Family members must identify what is expected of one another. Parents provide positive role models by not eating a lot of junk food. You follow diet guidelines and expected patterns of behavior in order to balance your diabetes. Learn to identify the stresses within your family.

Changes for Your Parents

Your parents probably experienced a lot of the same emotions you did when they learned you had diabetes: denial, anger, and guilt. Your mother may feel she should have done something else while she was pregnant with you or she should have fed you different food. No one is responsible for diabetes. You may find that your parents are overprotective. They may take on the responsibility of monitoring and treating your diabetes. At the doctor's office, they may be the ones to ask the questions and get all the answers. While this is all right for the first few months after diagnosis, it is not the way for you to learn to be responsible for yourself.

If your mother or father is talking to the doctors without you, ask that you be allowed to sit in. Remind them that it is your disease and that you need to know all you can. Your parents may be afraid that too much information will frighten you or that you won't understand what the doctor is saying. You can remind them that the more information a person has about an illness, the easier it is to come to terms with it and control it.

Sometimes parents react to learning a child has diabetes with pessimism. If you hear your parents saying things like "Oh, John will never live a normal life" or "Poor Mary, she'll never grow up to have any children," your first reaction may be to believe them. Don't. You know that with proper care you can control your diabetes and live a relatively normal life and have children. If your parents express negative thoughts about your illness, talk to them. Tell them that what they say makes you feel bad. They are probably not aware that what they are saying is having any effect on you. They aren't saying things to be mean, but rather because they love you and are frightened. If necessary, ask your health care provider to talk to them and give them more information. The key to understanding and coping with anything is knowledge. The more people know about something, the easier it is for them to deal with it, diabetes included.

Some teenagers try to punish their parents by doing things that they know they shouldn't do. The important thing to remember is that if you are doing things that have an impact on your diabetes, you could do harm to yourself that you will have to live with for the rest of your life. Proper care for diabetes starts immediately. There is no time off!

Your Siblings

Brothers and sisters will probably experience the same feelings that you and your parents do but with some other feelings as well. While they may accept the initial extra attention that your diagnosis focuses on you, after a while they may begin to resent it. They may feel that your mother or father is neglecting them, that somehow you have become more special and more important to everyone than they are. They may act out and say mean, hateful things to you as a way of expressing their resentment. They may accuse you of deliberately getting sick in order to get all the attention.

Although it may feel good to be the center of attention for a while, this can cause other problems in the family. You will always have diabetes, but you will not always be a child or a teenager. If you and other family members belong to a diabetes support group, this is an issue that could be addressed during a support meeting. Maybe other members could help your parents understand that too much attention is not good for the rest of the family. And too much attention is not good for you either. You need to be developing the skills you will need as an adult. After all, you don't really want your parents to take care of you forever, do you?

Sometimes having diabetes means that you have to grow up and accept more responsibility sooner than you or your family had planned. You may be the one who has to take the initiative for things. If your siblings are acting out because you have diabetes, try and tell your parents your concerns about what is happening within the family. Be honest about how you feel. Ask them to help you talk with your siblings. If your parents are not responsive, then you can make it easier by showing your brother or sister more attention yourself. Try to understand that they don't mean the careless things they say.

When a child, no matter how old, is diagnosed with a disease, it is natural for other family members to rally

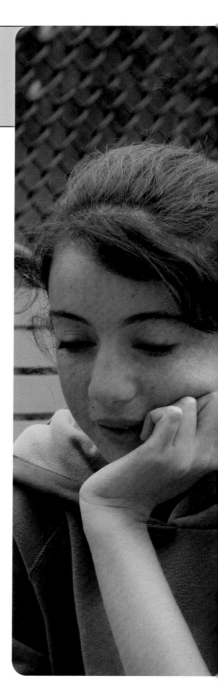

A sibling or a friend can make a great support base if you find yourself worried or afraid in the wake of a diabetes diagnosis.

around that child to give comfort and aid. But it is important to remember that other members of the family continue to need attention, affection, and comfort as well. While a sick person may require a lot of care, it doesn't mean that others, especially young children, will understand.

When someone is diagnosed with diabetes, it's time for the family to develop a support network. Other family members, teachers, and health care professionals can and should work together to provide support not only for the person with diabetes but for all members of the family.

Younger brothers and sisters may worry that diabetes is contagious and may stay away from you. Explain to them that germs do not cause diabetes, so they

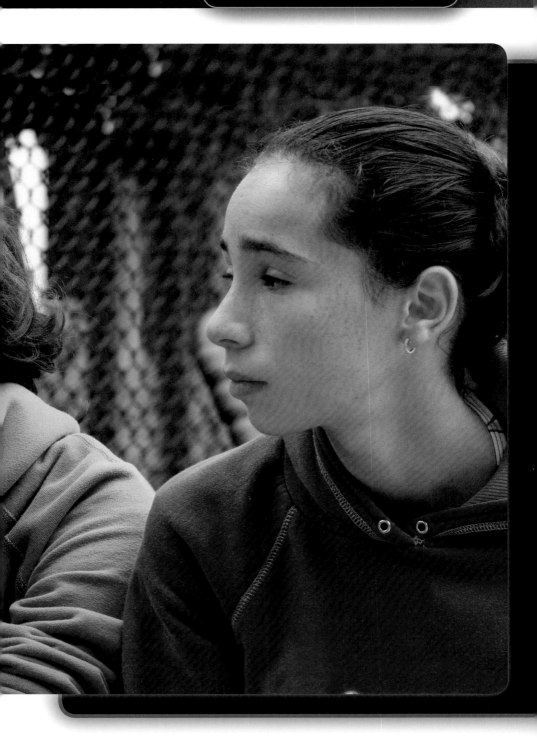

cannot get it by being close to you. Encourage them to help you in your daily care. Let them watch you do a finger stick or give yourself insulin. This may take some of their fear away. If they are old enough, you might even let them do the finger stick for you.

Sometimes brothers or sisters may fear getting the disease, not because it's contagious but because they know that heredity plays a part in determining who gets diabetes. Brothers and sisters of someone with diabetes have a 10 percent chance of getting the disease. If you sense that is what's going on, try to be a role model for them so that they lose some of their fear. Talk to them about what it is like having diabetes.

CHAPTER 5

It is normal not to want others to know about your diabetes at first. You may need time to think about what having diabetes means to you before sharing your diagnosis with your friends. But after a while, keeping your diabetes a secret may become an unnecessary burden to you, your family, and your friends. Although you do not have to tell everyone you have diabetes, there are several people you should tell.

You should tell your teachers and your school administrators. You should let your school know that you have diabetes so that if you have sick days you will be able to make up your schoolwork without a problem. You should also tell people at your school so that there is not a problem when you carry syringes to school. You should tell your teachers so that they will understand when you have to test during class or give yourself an injection, or if you need to eat a snack. Telling your teachers in advance will avoid problems later on. If your teachers are not understanding, you can have your doctor or another member of your health care team speak to them. You also need to tell your teachers so that they can be aware of the signs of hypoglycemia or hyperglycemia and be prepared to react if either of those conditions arise.

If you are involved in sports, you should tell your coach. Because exercise has an effect on

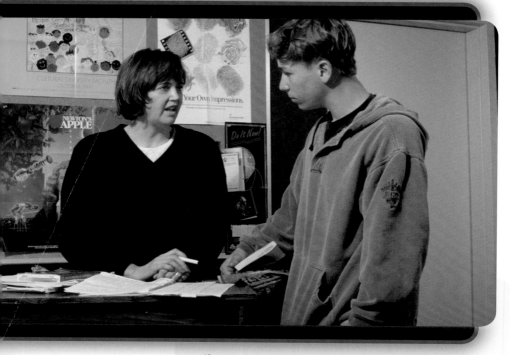

If you discover that diabetes is affecting your work in school, be proactive and talk to a teacher or school counselor about finding ways to keep your studies on track.

glucose levels, your coach needs to be aware of potential problems, just as your teachers do, so that he or she can react to them in time. If you are afraid to tell your coach because you think you will not be allowed to participate, you may want to talk to someone in the school administration first. There is no reason to prevent students who have their diabetes in control from participating in athletic activities. People with diabetes can be found in every type of sport today.

There is no real need to tell your classmates, but if you are testing during class, they will probably figure it out. Letting your classmates know you have diabetes and answering their questions about the disease are good ways to educate others.

You should tell your friends. You want your friends to know that you have diabetes for several reasons. Keeping your diabetes a secret from your friends means that you will have to waste a lot of time making up stories about why you can't eat that extra dessert or free order of fries.

Keeping your diabetes a secret means that you will have to keep all of your testing supplies and insulin hidden while you are at school and whenever your friends come over to your house. Keeping your diabetes a secret means that if you get into trouble with your diabetes, no one will know what is happening and, worse, no one will be able to help you. Keeping your diabetes a secret will add to the stress in your daily life, and you know that too much stress is not good for a person with diabetes.

Another reason to tell your friends about your diabetes and to explain to them what it means to have diabetes is that one of the signs of hypoglycemia is irritability. If you appear cranky all of a sudden when you are usually upbeat, a friend who knows about diabetes may be more understanding and may even alert you to the fact that you need to test your blood sugar. A friend may save your life someday.

If you are reluctant to tell someone about having diabetes, ask yourself why. Are you afraid that person will not like you anymore? In some cases, someone you tell will begin to avoid you. There is not much you can do about that except realize the person was probably not a good friend after all. While that may not make you feel better at first, later you'll see that you have friends who are loyal and you can trust.

Are you afraid that person will treat you differently if he or she knows you have diabetes? When you tell someone you have diabetes, you should also give that person some information about the disease. When you first tell someone, he or she may ask all sorts of questions. That is a natural response. Answer questions as honestly as you can. Be certain to let people know that having diabetes does not mean that you are a different person. Having diabetes means that you have to balance diet and exercise, not retire from your social life.

Are you ashamed of having diabetes? It is important to remember that diabetes is a disease that anyone can get. Diabetes does not mean that a person is good or bad. Having diabetes does not mean that you lose your identity. Do not let the fact that you have diabetes make you feel that you are somehow different. You aren't.

Your School Administrators and Teachers

Your teachers and the school nurse need to receive as much information as possible about diabetes and about your experience with diabetes. Don't presume that

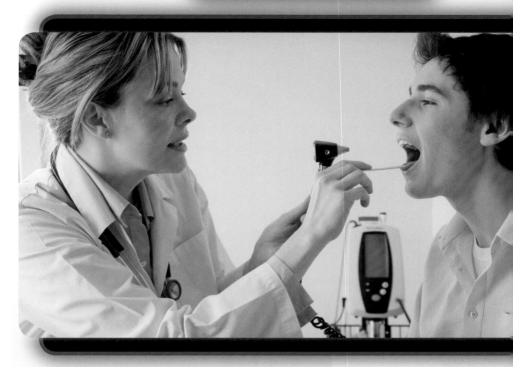

Your school nurse is a good go-to adviser when it comes to handling diabetes in school. Talk to him or her about your finger stick tests and the best place for you to perform them.

anyone already knows all about diabetes. There may be some basic misconceptions and fears that you and your parents can correct by providing current information. If you have special needs, then your teachers need to know about them. You may carry food such as orange juice or cheese and crackers in case of an insulin reaction. You may need to have a snack in the middle of a class when there is a rule that no eating is allowed. You have a right to expect the school to be flexible with its rules in order to accommodate your special needs. You may have to get written permission from your doctor to perform finger sticks and to take insulin while you are at school.

Different schools may have different rules. Some schools may allow you to perform finger sticks in the classroom while others may require that you go to the nurse's office or the bathroom. Also, unless your parents request it, you do not need a nurse to be present while you perform a finger stick or inject insulin. No matter where you do finger sticks or inject insulin, be sure to carry some sort of container to put the lancets and syringes in so that you can dispose of them properly. Diabetes is not contagious, but someone could get a serious infection if he or she accidentally got stuck with a used lancet or syringe. Be considerate of others.

Make certain the proper school officials are aware that you inject insulin and need to use a syringe. With today's high incidence of substance abuse in schools, you do not want to be wrongly accused of using drugs. Even though everyone would eventually realize a mistake had been made, you would have been subjected to an unnecessarily stressful situation. Try to get all of this information straight before there is a problem at school.

DIABETES AND ATHLETICS

Every day does not have to be a fight for your rights, but if something is really important to you, then you have to stand up for yourself. It is not always easy to be assertive, but with practice, it becomes easier.

If you are involved in athletics, make certain your coach or physical education teacher can recognize the difference between hypoglycemia (low blood sugar) and hyperglycemia (high blood sugar). If your coach or physical education teacher doesn't know very much about diabetes, take some time to share the information you have. Teach him or her how to give and read a glucose test. This is important for him or her to know anyway. Sometimes the best approach is to educate rather than wait until an incident occurs.

You have a right to be accepted by teachers and peers. In return, the school and your teachers have a right to expect you to be honest about your condition and to provide them with the information necessary to help them care for you in the event of an emergency.

If people in your school are not respectful of your rights, they may be guilty of discrimination. Your school does not have a right to require that you take your insulin only before or after class. If you can do it at those times, that is terrific, but if you can't, you have a right to inject your insulin whenever you are supposed to do it. Your school does not have the right to prevent you from eating a necessary snack. Your school does not have the right to prevent you from making up work missed because of sick days.

Schools have something called the 504 plan that allows students to request accommodation due to missed days. This means that your school is required to allow you to make up work missed without penalty. The 504 plan protects students who are considered to have "a disability in one of life's functions." The wide fluctuation in blood sugar is an impairment to a life function. Also, your school should have a "Health Impaired" section under its special education rules that allows you to make up missed work.

Occasionally schools have problems with diabetic students who use the condition as an excuse to cut class. If your school has had this problem, you may find that the teacher is unwilling to work with you to help you manage your diabetes. If that is the case, there are several things you can try. First, remind the teacher that you are not that problem student and that each student should be judged on a case-by-case basis. Remind your teacher that diabetics are individuals, just like any other group of people. People with diabetes share a disease, not personalities or habits. If your teacher is not persuaded, ask someone on your health care team to call your school. If this is unsuccessful, there are legal options.

Changes for Classmates

If your classmates are aware that you have diabetes, they may ask you questions about it. Some of the questions will be about taking insulin. Questions such as "Does it hurt?" "How can you stand taking those shots every day?" "Aren't you afraid that you'll stick yourself in the wrong place?"

There are many summer camps for young people with diabetes. Some of these camps are for those who want to play a particular sport or for those who live in a certain area. There are camps just for girls and camps just for boys. Ask someone on your health care team for addresses or contact the ADA for information on camps.

At camp you will be with others who have similar problems to your own. Camp is a good place to learn more about diabetes and how to maintain control of it. It is also a great place to make friends with people who already understand most of what you are going through and who can share experiences with you. Camp is also a place where all the campers have diabetes themselves, so everyone can be more open with each other. Sometimes it just feels good to be able to relax and have fun and not have to explain about having diabetes.

CAMPS FOR PEOPLE WITH DIABETES

Some of these questions are the very same ones you asked when you first learned you had diabetes. The best approach to these questions is to answer truthfully. Usually that is the end of it. It is possible that you will have a classmate who is not very sensitive and who keeps asking you questions that become annoying. Or you may have a classmate who doesn't really know that much about diabetes and repeats many of the myths in order to hurt your feelings or make you angry.

The first thing you should do is to talk to your friends. Friends are there to listen to you. If someone hurts your feelings, talking to your friends may be helpful. They may be able to offer solutions or help by just listening and taking your side. It is important to have a support network of teachers, friends, and family. It is also important to use that network in times of stress. Having your feelings hurt by an insensitive classmate creates stress, and stress can alter glucose levels.

Another thing you can do is to learn to stand up for yourself. This isn't always easy. Being assertive can be very difficult or frightening. But if you know that you are being treated unfairly or that hurtful things are being said about you, stand up for yourself. Explain yourself to that person. This may or may not help the person understand your situation, but the important thing is that you have asserted yourself. When you do that, you increase your self-esteem. You know that you did everything you could to solve the problem.

Sometimes being assertive doesn't work. If that is the case, you may have to turn to others for help. Talk to your teachers or the school guidance counselor. They may be able to give suggestions on how to handle difficult people and take care of yourself at the same time. It may seem unfair that you should have to be the one to find a solution, but that's part of growing up and becoming a responsible adult. Remember, you are not alone. You have friends and family to comfort you, and you have teachers and other people at school to intervene for you if you need them to. Most of all, you have yourself, and you are learning just how strong you are each and every day.

CHAPTER 6

Before the discovery of insulin, diabetes was a fatal disease. Although advances in medical science have allowed people with diabetes to live long and healthy lives, there is still no cure, and diabetics still face an increased risk for other health problems. Over a long period of time, diabetes can cause problems with your eyes, kidneys, heart, feet, skin, and nerves. What you do now to take care of yourself can affect your future. Keeping yourself healthy will decrease your risk of developing some of these conditions, but you should still know the risks that every person with diabetes faces.

EYES

People with diabetes need to take good care of their eyes by having regular eye exams. Nearsightedness is a common eye problem that occurs in people with diabetes. A person who is nearsighted, or who has myopia (another name for nearsightedness), has trouble seeing things at a distance but can usually see things that are close. Nearsightedness occurs when high glucose levels cause different body chemicals to accumulate in the lens of the eye. This causes the lens to swell slightly and can cause vision blurriness. This is usually a temporary problem that can come and go with fluctuations in

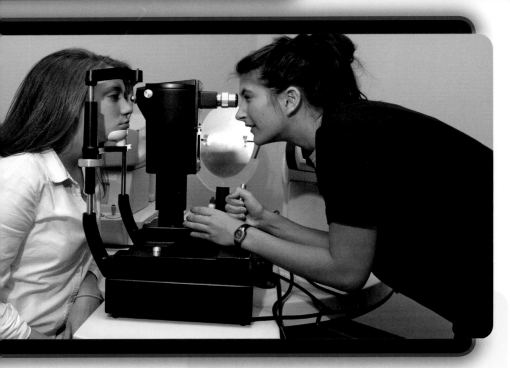

Your ophthalmologist can help monitor your eyes for any changes caused by your diabetes. Be sure to get a yearly eye exam so that any changes can be noted.

blood sugar levels and does not always mean you need glasses. But, if you experience this and go for an eye exam, be sure to mention that you have diabetes and that your glucose levels have been going up and down. Your eye doctor, or ophthalmologist, may recommend waiting a little while until your blood sugar stabilizes before determining if you need glasses.

A more serious eye disease is diabetic retinopathy. This occurs when the small vessels in the back of the eye break and cause damage to the retina. Diabetic retinopathy is the major contributor to blindness in the United States. Controlling your blood sugar can prevent this.

Researchers have found that keeping your blood pressure under control can also reduce the risk of diabetic retinopathy. Seventy percent of people with type 1 diabetes eventually develop this complication. Because this disease can develop rapidly during puberty no matter what type of diabetes you have, it is extremely important to have regular eye checkups every year. If your blood sugar is under control, chances are your vision is very good. Blurry vision can be a symptom of hypoglycemia or hyperglycemia, not necessarily eye disease. You can have diabetic retinopathy and still have good vision. Fortunately, there are things that can be done to prevent blindness in people diagnosed with diabetic retinopathy. Laser surgery can reduce the loss of vision by up to 60 percent in the early stages. If you have any problem with your sight, no matter how minor it may seem, it is best to see your doctor. Early detection is the key, so don't hesitate to have a checkup even if you don't have any symptoms.

People with diabetes are also at greater risk for cataracts (a condition in which the lens clouds up and looks milky), open-angle glaucoma (the most common form of glaucoma), and neovascular glaucoma (which mainly appears to affect people with diabetes). Teens with type 1 diabetes and poor glucose level control can develop "snowflake," or metabolic cataracts. This problem is frequently improved by carefully controlling glucose levels. Glaucoma is caused by increased pressure within the eye, which, if left untreated, can damage the back of the eye. This damage, in turn, will cause vision loss, headaches, and eye pain. Open-angle glaucoma is commonly treated with medical or laser surgery and usually results in a decrease in pressure within the eye and normalization of vision. Open-angle glaucoma is a disease that usually occurs in older people. The older you are and the longer you have had diabetes, the greater your chances of developing this disease. Neovascular glaucoma is a very severe form of glaucoma that usually develops in people who suffer from severe diabetic retinopathy. This disease can be treated with laser surgery if discovered early enough.

All of these diseases can be treated if detected early enough. Don't wait until you have a problem to see an ophthalmologist or retinologist. Remember, warning signs don't always occur with or precede these eye diseases, so make certain that an eye specialist is a part of your health care team.

TEETH

Diabetes does not cause cavities, nor does it increase your chances of having cavities. But people with diabetes are more prone to gum disease or periodontal disease if their glucose levels are not relatively stable. Remember, high glucose levels make it more difficult for the body to fight infection. Periodontal disease can cause gum loss and eventually tooth loss. Smoking also increases the risk of periodontal disease. Tooth loss makes it difficult to chew food and thus may discourage proper nutrition.

Teeth that come out as a result of periodontal disease cannot be replaced. Because periodontal disease damages the gums, dentures will not fit properly, and, again, this will discourage proper dietary habits. It is very important to maintain good dental hygiene at home by brushing and flossing daily and to have regular dental checkups at least every six months.

KIDNEYS

Diabetics of either type are more prone to kidney and bladder infections than other people. Infection can cause tissue damage to the kidneys over a period of time. This damage is called diabetic nephropathy and can lead to end-stage renal disease. End-stage renal disease occurs when a person's kidneys have lost their ability to function. A person with end-stage renal disease needs to have kidney dialysis or a kidney transplant to stay alive. In the United States, people diagnosed with end-stage renal disease often have diabetes. High blood pressure increases the chances of developing this disease. If you have type 2 diabetes and smoke cigarettes or have high cholesterol levels, you further increase your risk for this disease. Controlling your blood sugar and your blood pressure as well as practicing good health habits can prevent or delay kidney complications. In addition, any urinary tract infection should be treated immediately. Your doctor should perform a urinalysis every year to determine the potential for this disease. At present there is no cure for end-stage renal disease.

NERVOUS SYSTEM

Diabetes can cause negative changes in the nervous system (neuropathy). These changes may feel like a tingling or buzzing. Hands and feet may become numb. You may not be able to tell the difference between hot and cold. As with most other diabetes complications, risk for diabetic neuropathy increases if you have poor blood glucose control, smoke, drink alcohol, or have hypertension. You can lessen your chances of developing diabetic neuropathy by maintaining a healthy weight, exercising regularly, not smoking, and keeping your diabetes under control.

LEGS AND FEET

It is very important to take extra care of your feet and legs. Diabetes can damage the nerves and cause problems with the blood flow in these areas. If you have some sort of nerve damage in your feet or legs, you may not be able to feel if something is happening to those areas, so check them daily (don't forget to check between your toes) and follow these sensible care instructions.

Wash your feet daily with warm water and soap. Be sure to wash between your toes. Dry your feet thoroughly, especially between your toes. This is where athlete's foot grows. Use a lotion on dry skin (but not between your toes!). Change your socks every day. When your shoes begin to wear out or get dirty, wash them or replace them, whichever is necessary. (Stinky sneakers aren't

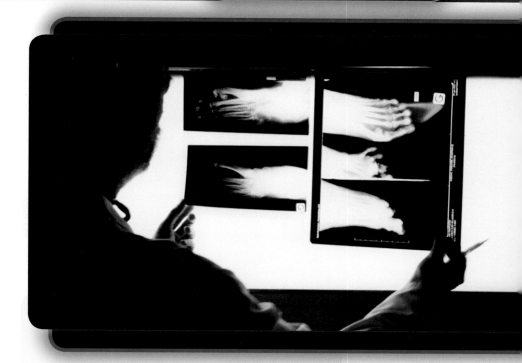

A doctor checks the X-rays of a diabetes patient for infections. Learning to take good care of your feet is one of the most important things you must learn to do after being diagnosed with diabetes.

cool, even if you don't have diabetes. There are a variety of odor-eating pads that you can buy to help tone down sneaker odor. Usually the odor develops because the sneakers never have time to dry out between use.) Try to alternate your shoes so you don't wear the same pair every day. Always wear shoes; don't go barefoot. Check the insides of your shoes before you put them on. That way you won't accidentally cut yourself on a pebble or something that found its way into your shoe. Wear flip-flops in the gym or in public swimming pools.

ASK DR. JAN, PSYCHOLOGIST

First name: Arianna

Question:
My friend has type 1 diabetes, and she is on insulin and never takes it, which I know can destroy her body. How can I talk to my friend about the serious effects of not taking her insulin?

Answer:
Type 1 diabetes, sometimes referred to as juvenile diabetes or childhood diabetes, is a condition where the person's body does not produce insulin. People with type 1 diabetes must take insulin to live. Type 2 diabetes usually occurs in individuals who have been in poor physical condition and overweight for some period of time. You might be surprised to learn that it is common for patients, particularly with type 2 diabetes, to be resistant to taking insulin shots even though their doctors insist upon it. Some studies show that as many as 72 percent of patients are reluctant to use insulin at first (*British Medical Journal*, 1995). There are several reasons that patients give for not wanting to take their insulin shots, including fear of needles and a resistance to accepting the diagnosis of diabetes.

Consider asking your friend why she is unwilling to take her insulin. If she doesn't believe that she has diabetes, offer to go with her to her doctor so that she can discuss it further. If she's afraid of needles, it might be necessary for her to return to her doctor for additional training until she is more comfortable with it. If she's still too afraid, she can work with a mental health professional trained in systematic desensitization, a behavioral technique that helps patients get over fears that interfere with their functioning. Most important, let her know how much you care about her and that you will help support her in addressing this challenge. If she refuses after all of your efforts, consider speaking to her parents, who may not be aware that she is not taking her insulin. Even though this can be difficult to do, your friend's health will be at risk if she doesn't take proper care of herself. Sometimes being a true friend means doing what's necessary, even if it's not easy.

Ask a Question

Do you have a question that you would like answered? E-mail your question to Dr. Jan at drjan@rosenpub.com. If your question is selected, it will appear on the Teen Health & Wellness Web site in "Dr. Jan's Corner."

If you have an urgent question on a health or wellness issue, we strongly encourage you to call a hotline to speak to a qualified professional or speak to a trusted adult, such as a parent, teacher, or guidance counselor. You can find hotlines listed in the For More Information section of this book, or at www. teenhealthandwellness.com/static/hotlines.

Now many people wear special shoes for swimming, so you won't look any different from anyone else.

Avoid anything that restricts circulation, such as crossing your legs or wearing tight shoes, stockings, socks, or tights. If you can't find comfortable socks or stockings, there are specialty stores that carry socks, stockings, and other apparel especially for people who have diabetes. Most of the clothing looks just like regular clothing. It usually is just not as tight fitting. If you have an ingrown toenail, corn, or callus, go to a podiatrist so he or she can properly treat your feet. Don't try to play doctor! Let a professional help you. Check your feet and legs every day for cracks in the skin or cuts or sores. If something looks unusual, don't hesitate to call your health care provider or podiatrist.

Smoking cigarettes increases the risk of damage to the nerves in the feet. If the nerves in your legs or feet are damaged, you may not be able to feel a cut or sore there, and it could get worse. Infections and poor blood flow are the major reasons for amputations in diabetics.

HEART

People with diabetes face an increased risk of developing heart problems. High glucose levels contribute to the risk of heart disease by increasing the potential for clogged arteries. Clogged arteries limit blood flow to the heart. The risk of heart disease increases even more if you smoke, have high blood pressure, use certain drugs, or have high cholesterol levels. You can lessen your chances of developing heart disease by eating a balanced diet, maintaining a healthy weight, exercising regularly, not smoking, and keeping your diabetes under control. Your doctor should check your blood pressure at each visit.

SKIN

If your diabetes is not properly controlled, you may become dehydrated, causing your skin to become very dry and itchy. Try using a lanolin-based cream or moisturizer. Don't put lotion between your toes. You want that area to remain

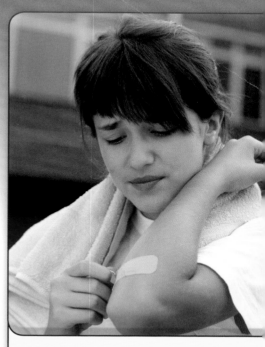

Even the most minor cuts can lead to serious infection when you have diabetes. Be sure to clean the cut well and monitor it carefully.

dry. If you find the skin between your toes getting too dry and cracking, consult your doctor. If you are having trouble controlling your diabetes, you need to watch out for skin infections. High blood glucose levels interfere with the action of bacteria-fighting cells. If you get a sore or a small cut anywhere, treat it immediately. Keep the area clean and watch it. If it does not heal within ten days, call your doctor. You may need an antibiotic.

CHAPTER 7

MAINTAINING YOUR HEALTH

Diabetes is not a simple disease. Remember that it is not really one disease but several diseases. Diabetes is complicated, but the more you learn about it, the better you will be able to cope with it. When you were first diagnosed with diabetes, you or your parents were given some basic information and procedures necessary to survive on a day-to-day basis. That information included how to put insulin into a syringe, how to inject insulin, how to care for your diabetes equipment, and how to monitor your blood sugar and ketone levels with finger sticks and urine tests. You probably were given information on nutrition and diet. After you start taking control of your diabetes, you will find there is much more to learn, from simple hygiene needs to information about sophisticated equipment, such as insulin infusion pumps and oral medications.

DIABETES MANAGEMENT AND TESTING

Testing is important because you need to know if your diabetes is being controlled. When blood sugar levels are too high and insulin is too low, the cells are not getting the fuel they need to function properly. As a young person, you need your cells to function as close to normal as possible in order to maintain normal growth and development. Monitoring your blood sugar and ketones is one way to help yourself. Finger sticks and urine tests are short-term tests. That means the tests give you an indication of what is happening right now. The tests cover a short period of time. You should do self-monitoring of glucose (SMBG) at least four times a day to ensure that you are controlling your diabetes.

The two short-term tests you should do are the finger stick and the urine test. You can do both of these yourself at home or at school.

Finger Stick Test

The finger stick test involves pricking yourself with a finger stick, or lancet (like a pin), to get a drop of blood. This blood sample is then either compared to a chart or inserted into a machine called a glucose monitor. Both of these methods will determine your glucose level.

Take readings in sequence before meals and at bedtime to see if your blood sugar is following a normal pattern throughout the day. This also helps determine if you and your health care team have found the proper balance between insulin, exercise, and diet to suit your individual needs. The ideal is to keep blood sugar levels between 80 and 180 mg/dl. The normal blood sugar level for a person without diabetes is between 70 and 120 mg/dl before meals and less than 180 mg/dl two hours after eating.

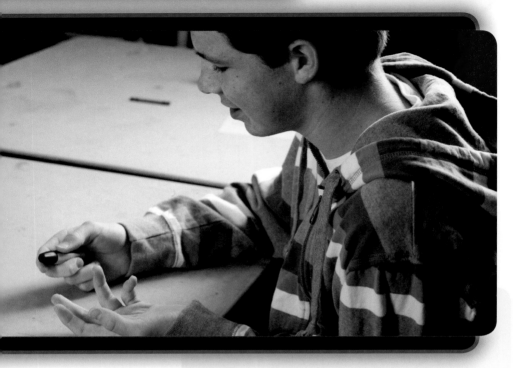

Blood sugar testing may be a daunting task at first—especially if you are afraid of needles! But after you become accustomed to it, you may find that it's not as painful as you originally thought.

Urine Tests

Urine testing is done to measure ketones. You do this the first time you urinate in the morning, every morning. Urine testing is not as reliable as testing your blood. Urine tests rely on the renal threshold. This is the level at which your kidneys begin to "spill" sugar into your urine. It is not uncommon in young people for urine to show high levels of sugar in the blood when in fact the amount is really OK for that person. Also, urine tests only measure for high blood sugar and can't show low blood sugar (hypoglycemia). The finger stick and urine tests can show the following results:

- Negative sugars, negative ketones: this means that your blood sugar stayed between 80 and 180 mg/dl overnight. This is what you want to see.
- Negative sugars and positive ketones: negative sugars indicate that your blood sugar remained below 180 mg/dl overnight, but the positive ketones mean you may have had a low blood sugar reaction while you were sleeping.
- Positive sugars and negative ketones: this indicates that your blood sugar probably went over 180 mg/dl during the night.
- Positive sugars and positive ketones: this means that your overnight blood sugar went over 180 mg/dl and that your diabetes is out of control. Call your health care professional immediately.

Chemstrip K and Ketostix are the brand names of two commonly used ketone testing strips.

If you use insulin, you should test for ketones whenever you have two glucose readings in a row that are above 200 mg/dl. Both type 1 and type 2 diabetics should test whenever they get sick, have an infection, or experience extra stress.

It's natural to get tired of testing every day and to find that testing gets you down. It is OK to take a break now and then if you think it will get you motivated again. But you need to be careful. Don't decide to take a break from testing the same day you decide to go out for the football team or eat an extra snack. Any change from your regular routine means that you need to test yourself so that you can modify your insulin intake to keep in balance. If you find that you need a break every few days, that's not good. Daily testing is something that is or should be a part of your life. It is something you must do every day to ensure your health. You can't just let it go. If you find it too much of a bother, you need to talk with someone, either a member of your health care team, a counselor, or someone you know who also has diabetes. While it is OK to skip a test now and then, it is not OK to skip a day or two. At the very least, you must test four times a day at least three times a week.

WHAT ARE HYPOGLYCEMIA AND HYPERGLYCEMIA?

What if your blood sugars are way off the mark? Is it your fault that you have bad blood sugars? First of all, when your blood sugar doesn't fall within the desired range, it doesn't mean that you are at fault. Nor does it mean that you have "bad" blood sugar. Try not to think in terms of good and bad. When your blood sugar doesn't fall within the desired range, it means just that: it is not within the desired range.

The response should never be guilt; it should be to recognize that the proportions between diet, insulin, and exercise have to be redesigned to achieve balance again.

Balance is always your goal, not guilt. Remember, the hormones associated with puberty can have an effect on glucose levels. It is possible to experience a change in your blood sugar levels even if you are doing all the right things. You may have to remind your parents about this as well.

What Is Hypoglycemia?

Hypoglycemia, commonly called low blood sugar or insulin reaction, happens when the blood glucose level drops below 70 mg/dl. It generally happens quickly. Hypoglycemia can happen for a variety of reasons that you may be able to control, such as too much insulin, not eating enough food, skipping a snack or meal, or engaging in a lot of unexpected exercise.

You can avoid hypoglycemia caused by insufficient food or missing a meal by carrying a snack with you at all times. If you are in a position where you have no choice but to engage in extra exercise, be certain to check your glucose level as soon as you can. But hypoglycemia may occur for no apparent reason, and you have no control over that.

If a person loses consciousness and cannot ingest food to bring his or her glucose level up, glucagon, available only through a prescription, can be injected to raise the glucose level quickly. Family members should be trained to be on the lookout for signs of hypoglycemia and know when and how to inject glucagon.

The symptoms of hypoglycemia are trembling, tingling lips, irritability, mood swings, sweating, hunger,

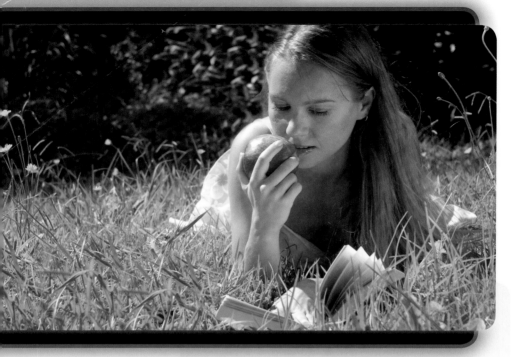

If you suffer from hypoglycemia, always carry a healthy snack along just in case. An apple or another piece of fruit can make a healthy, and portable, snack.

fatigue, paleness, and loss of coordination. A person with hypoglycemia may also appear to be drunk. If you are with a friend who knows the symptoms, he or she will know you are suffering from hypoglycemia. But because you can't always be with people you know, hypoglycemia is a good reason to wear a medical alert bracelet. If you are somewhere where you don't know anyone and you develop hypoglycemia, people may assume you are intoxicated and do nothing to help you. Worse, you could be in a situation where police assume you are drunk and arrest you rather than try to help you. To treat hypoglycemia, you need a fast-acting sugar.

There are several commercial products available that your doctor may recommend you keep close at hand. Hypoglycemia can also be treated with fruit juice, raisins, or hard candy. The benefits of commercial glucose tablets are that they work faster than candy, have fewer calories, and usually contain no fat or sodium. Plus, you probably won't use them to cheat on your diet. Also, because the dosage is specific, unlike being told to take a few pieces of hard candy, you are less likely to push your blood glucose level up too high, which can happen if you rely on candy.

What Is Hyperglycemia?

Hyperglycemia is also called diabetic coma or high blood sugar. It comes on slowly as a result of rising blood sugar levels. The symptoms are fatigue, extreme thirst, and frequent urination. When ketones begin to develop, you may feel nauseated and start to vomit, have stomach cramps, and your breath may smell sweet. Some of the causes of hyperglycemia, such as forgetting to take your insulin or eating too much of the wrong foods, can be prevented.

Hyperglycemia is treated by adjusting insulin intake. If you notice any of these symptoms, check your glucose levels immediately. Sometimes people near you can smell the sweetness in your breath. Some people say it has a fruity smell. If someone mentions this to you, act immediately and monitor your glucose. Like hypoglycemia, hyperglycemia may occur no matter what you do. Hyperglycemia can develop into a coma if it is not caught in time. The best prevention is to monitor your glucose levels regularly, especially if you are not feeling well.

WHAT IS TIGHT CONTROL OF DIABETES?

Most people with diabetes follow a conventional approach to maintenance. That means that they test a couple of times a day, use the same insulin dosage each day, and see their doctor about four times a year. Tight control means more of everything. It means testing, at the very least, four times a day and adjusting insulin dosages accordingly, which means injecting insulin several times a day (multiple daily injections or MDIs) or using an insulin pump.

In the 1980s, the National Institutes of Health (NIH) began a study called the Diabetes Control and Complications Trial (DCCT). The purpose of the study was to determine if people with diabetes who could keep their blood glucose levels within normal ranges or near normal ranges could postpone or avoid future diabetes-related complications. When the study ended in 1993, the conclusion was a resounding yes. People with diabetes who can keep their blood glucose levels within normal ranges or near normal ranges can postpone or avoid future diabetic complications.

How Does Tight Control Work?

Tight control is also called intensive therapy. "Intensive" is the key word. Intensive therapy is meant to help a person with diabetes have a steady supply of insulin similar to that of a person without diabetes. Although practicing tight control over diabetes is a lot of work, it actually gives a person more freedom. Because the insulin is delivered in very small amounts, it can be adjusted to match a change in activity or diet. People who practice conventional therapy have to adjust what they are doing to match the insulin they have taken. Whether the person uses MDIs or an insulin pump to control the amount of insulin, he or she must monitor blood glucose levels often, adjust insulin dosages, maintain good records, and follow healthy diet and exercise guidelines. If you think you want to practice tight control, talk with your health care team. They can work out a plan for you. Tight control is a lot of work, so you may want to start slowly. You could begin right now by doing more frequent SMBGs and then working into MDIs. But you need to know that if you begin intensive therapy, you will probably gain some weight. In the DCCT study, people gained an average of ten pounds. Also, with intensive therapy, you do not have reservoirs of glucose to tap into in case of low blood sugar, or hypoglycemia. So you need to be aware of the symptoms and be prepared to treat them.

If you have type 2 diabetes, the keys to tight control are diet and exercise. You don't have to monitor your blood glucose levels as frequently, maybe only once a week or once a day. Remember, if you have type 2 diabetes, your body does not use insulin efficiently, so glucose remains in your bloodstream. Exercise helps lower glucose levels.

You are probably unprepared to practice tight control if you are still angry or depressed about having diabetes or if you are not willing to become an active member of your health care team and do all the necessary testing and record keeping. If you are not ready now, maybe you will be later on.

THE IMPORTANCE OF INSULIN

People with type 1 diabetes have to take insulin. When Leonard Thompson received the first insulin injection, it was very short-acting and had to be readministered frequently. Today there are better options. As with all types of medication, there are different types of insulin. In fact, there are more than thirty types of insulin. The trend is toward having all-human insulin products. Animal-based insulin comes from purified pork insulin and purified beef insulin. Animal-based insulin lasts longer than human insulin but may cause skin dents (lipoatrophies) or swelling (lipodystrophies) that human insulin does not seem to cause unless repeatedly injected into the same place. Lipoatrophies occur less often today because insulin manufacturers take extra precautions to assure the purity of their products.

Researchers originally hoped that human insulin would soon be available to everyone. Unfortunately human insulin isn't for everyone and there is a debate over the safety of human insulin products for some patients. Talk to your health care provider about any concerns you may have, and no matter what type of insulin you use, be certain to monitor your glucose levels on a regular schedule.

What Are the Types of Insulin?

These different types of insulin also vary in how quickly they act, how long they last, and how they look. You need to know not only the source of the insulin but its onset hours (how long it takes to get into the bloodstream and start working), its peak hours (how long it has its strongest effects in lowering blood sugar), and its duration hours (how long it stays in the bloodstream).

There is unmodified insulin, which gets into the bloodstream quickly and is clear and colorless. Rapid-acting insulin lasts six to eight hours. Lente insulin is made from beef, pork, or human insulin and contains zinc-insulin crystals. It reacts and looks like unmodified insulin but is used by people who have allergic reactions to unmodified insulin. Ultralente insulin is made from beef or human insulin and contains a lot of zinc, which causes the insulin to be absorbed more slowly and last longer than other types of insulin. Neutral protamine Hagedorn (NPH) insulins are made from beef, pork, human, or a combination of beef and pork insulin. NPH insulins contain an ingredient called protamine, which slows down insulin absorption but increases duration. NPH insulins are slower acting than unmodified insulin. They are a cloudy, milky suspension. Protamine zinc insulins (PZI) last thirty-six hours or more and are also cloudy, milky suspensions. Human insulin regular is clear and colorless. It looks like water. Human insulin NPH or lente is uniformly milk white.

All insulin bottles have a large letter or number on the label that indicates the kind of insulin it is. Regular (R) and semilente (S) insulin act quickly. NPH (N) and lente (L) are known as intermediate insulin. These insulins take a little longer to begin having an effect, but they last longer. Ultralente (U) is long-acting insulin, but its duration may depend upon the person. It takes even longer to start working than the other two types, but it lasts longer.

Most people use different types of insulin in order to maintain a consistent blood sugar level. Many people take a combination of insulin. Insulin that is 50/50 is half regular and half NPH. Insulin that is 30/70 is 30 percent regular insulin and 70 percent NPH insulin. There are also other combinations: 10/90, 20/80, and 40/60.

The first number indicates the percentage of regular insulin. Remember, R insulins are fast-acting. The second number indicates the percentage of intermediate-acting insulin. A 10/90 mixture means that the insulin is 10 percent R and 90 percent N.

These combinations give the user the benefit of fast action that lasts longer than if just using one or the other. Lente insulin is an intermediate-acting insulin that is made from three parts semilente and seven parts ultralente. Some insulins have other ingredients added to them to help prevent infections or to help them work longer. These additives affect how the insulin will work for you. Be certain to use the brand name, and not just the type, of insulin your doctor prescribes.

Your doctor will determine what kind of insulin works best for you depending on how much insulin your body produces, your diet, and your exercise habits. A new type of insulin is called insulin glargine (Lantus). It has a quick onset but is long-acting. Many type 1 patients use this at night to help prevent the dawn phenomenon.

When Do You Take Insulin?

You should set up a schedule to take your insulin at the same time or times every day. Because everyone is different, there is no definite rule about when to inject insulin. Your doctor or diabetes educator will help you decide when is best for you. It may be frightening, especially if you are afraid of needles, to think about injecting yourself with a syringe every day. With some time and practice, it won't be so frightening. Your doctors will show you how to inject insulin so that it is a relatively painless procedure.

If you are on a regular schedule, you reduce the risk of forgetting to inject your insulin. If you forget, as soon as you remember, test your blood glucose level and call a member of your health care team for advice.

How Do You Measure Insulin?

Insulin used to be measured by how much was required to change the blood glucose level in a rabbit. Today, the method is more sophisticated. Now insulin weight is based on a crystallized sample, and it is measured in units. When you buy insulin, the label on the bottle tells you how many units of insulin are in a cubic centimeter, or cc. (A centimeter is about as wide as the nail on your pinky finger.) The number of insulin units per cubic centimeter is called the concentration level. In the United States, the concentration level is almost always 100. That means there are 100 units of insulin per cc. This

Insulin Type	Onset Hours	Peak Hours	Duration Hours	Name
Short-acting	–	1 – 4	5 – 7	regular (R) semilente (S) insulin lispro (humalog)
Intermediate-acting	2 – 3	4 – 14	18 – 24	NPH (N) lente (L) human utralente (U) (depends on the person)
Long-acting	14 – 24	minimal	10 – 36	human ultralente (U) (depends on the person)

is written on the label as U-100. Syringes are usually marked in units of 1 cc. If you use a U-100 syringe and fill it with insulin, you are using 100 units of insulin, or 1 cc. If you fill it halfway, you are using 50 units, or 1/2 cc of insulin.

There are a variety of factors to consider before you decide what type or types of insulin you are going to use. Your lifestyle is a very important factor. As a teenager, you probably are very active and on the go a lot of the time. You may want to try different insulins or a combination of them. Your health care team will assist you in making a decision that is right for you.

How Do You Inject Insulin?

Insulin is injected because the digestive juices destroy it if it is taken orally. It is injected through the skin, not into a vein. Insulin eye drops and inhalers have both been produced, but right now the results are mixed. Some people inject insulin using a syringe, some people use an insulin pen injector, and others use a pump that automatically injects it. If you inject insulin, you should always have this equipment readily accessible:

- Insulin
- Syringe and needle
- Alcohol and sterile cotton
- Glucagon, in case of an emergency
- Test strips
- Medical identification

THE INSULIN RULES

- Always check the expiration date on the bottle. Never buy or use outdated insulin. Don't buy more insulin than you can use before the expiration date.

- Although it is unnecessary to keep insulin refrigerated, it is a good idea to keep it cool by storing it in the refrigerator. If you do not refrigerate your insulin, store it in a place free from excessive cold or heat. But don't store your insulin at room temperature. Don't freeze insulin. Check with your doctor or pharmacist about proper storage for your type of insulin.

- Don't shake the vials; roll them to mix the ingredients.

- Make sure the ingredients look the way they are supposed to. Regular insulin is clear. If it is cloudy or has particles in it, don't use it. If your insulin is supposed to be colorless and it has a yellow tint, don't use it. Also remember that insulin glargine, or Lantus, is also clear. Lente and NPH insulins look cloudy. If you see solid white particles stuck on the vial after you've rolled the vial, don't use it. If you see clumps of particles or crystals in the insulin, don't use it.

- Write down the name or type of insulin that you use, the species (beef, pork, or human), the company that makes it, the concentration (U-100), and the dosage. Memorize this. Keep a copy of it in your wallet or purse so that it's always handy. If you change types of insulin or dosages, remember to change this information on all of your medical records.

You should also change the site of the injection from time to time. Continually injecting into the same place can cause little lumps called lipodystrophies, also known as insulin-induced hypertrophy. Dents called lipoatrophies, also known as insulin-induced atrophy, can occur as well. Dents and lumps can also occur if you use impure animal-based insulins made from beef or pork. These lumps and dents are harmless, but you can lessen your chances of getting them by rotating your injection sites. One possibility is to use a different site for injections at different times. Make a rotation chart for injections. Some places most commonly used are the outer area of the upper arm; just below the hip bone in the upper buttock; above and below the waist avoiding a 2-inch (5-cm) circle around the navel; and the middle front of the thigh. You could use your thigh in the morning and your abdomen in the evening. Develop your own combination of injection sites for your chart. This way, while you are lessening the chances of lumps or dents, you are also maintaining a routine so that you know the timing and action of the insulin better than if you randomly changed the site daily.

Also remember: When you are injecting insulin just before physical activity, don't inject it into the area you will be using the most. In other words, if you are going to be running, don't inject insulin into your leg. It will absorb much faster than you are used to. Always wipe the top of the insulin vial with alcohol before you stick the needle in. Recap the needle when you are done. If you are using a coated needle, do not wipe it with alcohol.

The needle has a special coating that makes injections easier, and alcohol will remove this coating. As long as the needle has touched nothing but the vial and the injection site, you can use the needle again. Do not reuse the needle if you are mixing insulins or if it has touched anything other than the vial and the injection site. If your needles are not coated, you can sterilize them by boiling them. If you have questions about reusing needles and syringes, ask a member of your health care team for advice.

MEDICATIONS FOR TYPE 2 DIABETES

The most common therapy for people with type 2 diabetes is diet and exercise therapy. For some people, however, diet and exercise are insufficient to control their blood glucose levels. In those cases, the patients are given oral medications. There are four categories of these medications: alpha-glucosidase inhibitors, biguanides, sulfonylurea drugs, and thiazolidinediones. These medications may be prescribed alone, in combination with each other or other drugs, or with insulin.

The alpha-glucosidase inhibitor called acarbose (Precose) was approved by the Food and Drug Administration (FDA) in 1995. Acarbose lowers blood glucose levels by slowing down the digestion of carbohydrates.

The biguanide that you have probably heard about is called metformin, commonly sold under the trade

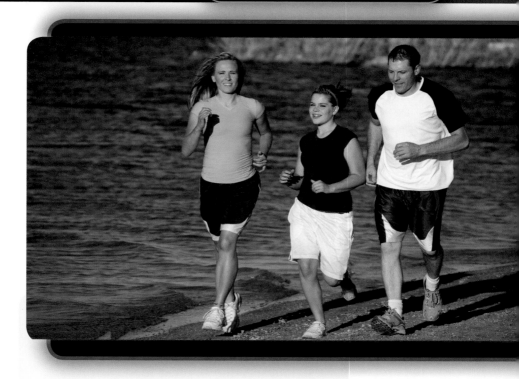

Exercise does not have to be strenuous to be effective. Going for a leisurely walk or a jog can be a fun way to get some exercise without hitting the gym.

name Glucophage. It was approved by the FDA in 1994. Metformin lowers blood sugar by helping the body to use insulin more effectively; it may work to help people with type 2 diabetes lose weight and consequently have lower cholesterol levels. For some people, the use of metformin may eliminate the need for insulin injections.

Sulfonylurea drugs have been around for a long time. These drugs are divided into two categories: first generation and second generation. First generation drugs are the first drugs that are used to treat a disease. The trade names of these drugs are Diabenese, Glucamide, Ronase, Tolinase, Orinase, Oramide, and Dymelor. Second generation drugs, such as Glucotrol, Diabeta, Glynase, Micronase, and Amaryl, are usually stronger and have fewer side effects than first generation drugs. Second generation drugs are not always effective for all people, so don't discount your doctor's advice if he or she suggests you use a first generation drug. All of these drugs work by helping the body to produce more insulin.

Your doctor and your health care team can help you determine which drug or drugs are best for you. Each medication has different side effects. One drug may be more effective for you than another.

If your doctor recommends that you try any of these drugs, remember that you still have to maintain your diet and exercise balance. None of these medications are a cure! Remember, the most common way doctors treat type 2 diabetes is through diet and exercise. In fact, if you take oral medication for type 2 diabetes and you regularly exercise and watch your diet, there may come a time when you no longer need medication. But never stop your medication without your doctor's advice.

CHAPTER 8

Diets for people with diabetes have changed drastically. In 1796, Dr. John Rollo's diet for people with diabetes was rancid milk, pork, suet, and bread. By the 1800s, people were told to take antimony, an element that induced vomiting and diarrhea. In the late 1800s, Dr. Arnoldo Cantani told his diabetic patients to fast every other day. Fortunately, things have changed a lot. The days of the diabetic diet are almost gone.

The fundamental key to good health—for anyone—is a good diet. This is especially true for people with diabetes. Although you can still eat the things you like, you must do so in moderation. Remember that part of everything you eat is turned into glucose. Because your body doesn't produce or use insulin effectively, you must be very careful to balance the amount of glucose you have and the amount of insulin you take. If you have type 2 diabetes, diet may be your main means of controlling the disease. Tight control for people with type 2 diabetes requires conscientious weight control. If you are seriously overweight, you need to eat low-calorie foods with high nutritional value to bring your weight within a healthy range.

Take your diet seriously. According to the ADA, most people with diabetes do not take their diets seriously. The purpose of a healthier

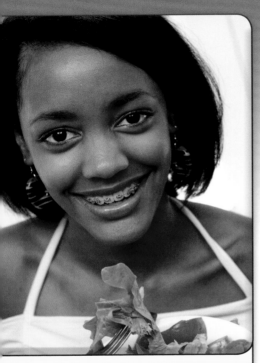

It can be difficult at first to adjust to a new way of eating. As you begin to make changes to your diet, you can seek advice from a dietician.

diet in the life of a person with diabetes is to control the blood glucose level. If you start taking care of your body now, you lessen the risks of many diabetes complications later in life. There are many ways to watch your diet. The following are three basic types of diet that most dietitians recommend:

1. **Weighed Diet.** With this type of diet, you have a specific menu with specific portions of specific foods. You have to weigh and measure all the foods you eat. Weight Watchers and many other weight-loss programs follow the weighed diet. It is not a bad idea to try this method out, even if you don't end up using it. That big bowl of cereal you have for breakfast each morning is probably three serving sizes. You will be surprised at the difference between your idea of a serving size and a "real" serving size. Ask your dietitian for a cookbook.

2. **Exchange Diet.** This type of diet is like the weighed diet. You still have to follow a diet plan using certain proportions, which means measuring your food. The difference is that you can mix and match your food.

If you are allowed to have one bread exchange at breakfast, you can have a slice of bread, a biscuit, or a cup of cereal. If your doctor puts you on an exchange diet, ask your dietitian for an exchange list.

3. **Free Diet.** This doesn't mean you can eat whatever you want. The free diet means you don't have to weigh your food, but you are expected to follow basic nutrition guidelines. This type of diet requires a lot of self-discipline.

THE ROLE OF SUGAR

Contrary to popular belief, sugar does not cause diabetes. Doctors used to warn people with diabetes to avoid sugar in the belief that a simple carbohydrate like sugar would raise the blood glucose levels much faster than a complex carbohydrate like bread. Recent studies have shown that simple and complex carbohydrates have the same effect on blood glucose levels in about the same amount of time. The ADA has released new diet guidelines for diabetics that do not limit the amount of sugar. That doesn't mean that you can now eat all the candy and drink all the soda you want. You must maintain your diet balance and remember that while simple and complex carbohydrates are absorbed at the same rate, they may not have the same nutritional value. Too much substitution of simple carbohydrates for complex carbohydrates could result in excess weight gain and loss of nutritional value. Remember that sugar is a carbohydrate, and too many carbohydrates can raise your blood glucose. It is not always easy to know what foods contain sugar even when looking at the label. Sugar is identified by many different names. Generally the names for sugar end in "ose," as in sucrose, but "carbohydrate" is the key word to look for. Carbohydrates are usually listed on food labels.

ADJUSTING TO A TYPE 1 DIABETES DIET

The three kinds of food that a person with type 1 diabetes can eat are divided into carbohydrates, proteins, and fats.

Carbohydrates

One hundred percent of a carbohydrate is turned into glucose. Carbohydrates are used for energy and have four calories per gram (.035 ounce) of weight. There are two kinds of carbohydrates: simple and complex.

Some examples of simple carbohydrates are candy, soda (nondiet), cookies, cakes, honey, and syrup. Some examples of complex carbohydrates are breads, potatoes, rice, cereal, pasta, vegetables, and some fruits.

Proteins

Proteins are used to repair cells and help us grow. Proteins contain four calories per gram of weight. Sixty percent of proteins break down into glucose. Protein is absorbed slowly by the body. Proteins come from all animal sources—meats, fish, and dairy products—and from nuts. Proteins can also be found in some plants and in grain. If you are having trouble with your kidneys because of diabetes, your doctor may recommend that you cut back on certain kinds of protein.

Fats

Fat has nine calories per gram of weight, and only 10 percent of it is turned into glucose. Fat is another source of energy for the body, but it must first be turned into ketones before it can be used. There are five kinds of fat, listed below.

Cholesterol

Cholesterol is not really a fat but is usually included in the list because it is similar to fat. Cholesterol has a very important relationship with fat because it is carried through the body in molecules of fat and protein called lipoproteins. The body uses cholesterol to build cell membranes and to help make certain hormones. Cholesterol is manufactured in the liver. In fact, all the cholesterol one needs is manufactured in the body. The other way to get cholesterol is from eating animal products such as meat and dairy products. You have probably heard that there are two kinds of cholesterol: good cholesterol (high-density cholesterol, or HDL) and bad cholesterol (low-density cholesterol, or LDL). The fact is that all cholesterol is the same. What makes cholesterol good or bad is the kind of lipoprotein that is used to transport it through the body.

High-density cholesterol is carried through the body by a lipoprotein that contains more protein than fat. This lipoprotein is called high-density lipoprotein, which is what HDL really is. HDL is called good cholesterol because it not only carries the necessary cholesterol through the body to the cells, but it then takes the leftover cholesterol and carries it back to the liver, where it can be broken down.

The other type of lipoprotein, called a low-density lipoprotein, is made up of more fat than protein. This is what LDL really is. LDL is called bad cholesterol because if there is too much LDL in the bloodstream or not enough HDL, the cholesterol still gets carried to the cells, but the LDL drops its excess cholesterol in the arteries instead of carrying it back to the liver. Different kinds of fats affect cholesterol levels in the body in different ways by raising or lowering the levels of LDL and HDL in the bloodstream.

Saturated Fat

Saturated fat usually comes from animals. The meat you eat contains saturated fat. Butter and whole milk are other examples of saturated fats. Too many saturated fats in a diet cause the liver to increase cholesterol production.

Monounsaturated Fat

Monounsaturated fats come mostly from plants and seafood. Examples are olive oil and canola oil. Monounsaturated fats are actually good for you in

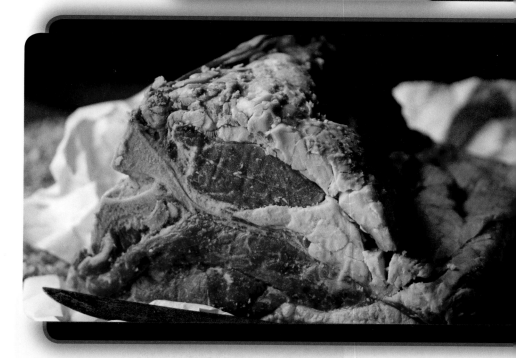

Red meat contains a lot of saturated fat. If you cannot cut it from your diet altogether, at least find ways to limit your red meat consumption to once or a few times per week.

moderation because they lower the levels of dangerous cholesterol in your bloodstream by increasing the HDL level.

Polyunsaturated Fat

Polyunsaturated fats are similar to monounsaturated fats in that they come from plants and seafood. But polyunsaturated fats lower not only the levels of LDL but the levels of HDL as well. Corn oil and safflower oil are examples of polyunsaturated fats.

Triglycerides

Triglycerides are another form of fat that people with diabetes have to pay special attention to, because high levels of triglycerides usually indicate a level of HDL that is too low or a level of LDL that is too high. Either one may mean increased risk for heart disease. Because a person with diabetes is already at risk, high levels of triglyceride may only increase it. The ADA recommends that people with diabetes follow these dietary guidelines:

1. Fats should be 30 percent or less of your daily calories.
2. Saturated fat should be 10 percent or less of your daily calories.
3. Protein should be between 10 and 20 percent of your daily calories.
4. Cholesterol should be 300 milligrams (.01 ounce) or less daily.
5. You should eat 20 to 35 grams (.70 to 1.23 ounces) of fiber a day.

Your health care team or dietitian can help you and your family come up with a meal plan that will work for all of you.

WHAT ARE YOU EATING?

Food labeling guidelines are quite helpful to people with diabetes. Look at the nutrition facts panel on the side of

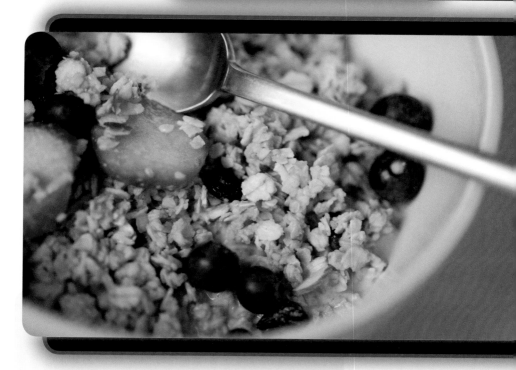

Be sure you check the nutrition information on your cereal box before pouring yourself a bowl. Limit yourself to one serving and keep track of the fat, fiber, and carbohydrate content you are consuming.

the food package. Check the daily values column that lists the percent of nutrients in that food. You want a food that has a low percentage of fats and cholesterol but a high percentage of fiber. If you have to monitor your daily intake of fat, the nutrition facts panel also gives you the total fat calories as well as the percentage of calories from fat. According to the ADA you should not get more than 30 percent of your daily calories from fat.

Carbohydrates and proteins are also listed. Another thing to watch for is the serving size. What you may think is a normal-size serving of cereal may actually be twice the product's serving size. Learn to weigh and measure your foods, especially if you have type 2 diabetes. The teenage years are a time when the body is growing rapidly, and teenagers generally need more food than adults do. The trick is to consume nutritious foods rather than just empty calories or calories that have no nutritional value.

YOUR EXERCISE REGIMEN

No matter what type of diabetes you have, your doctor will recommend that you exercise regularly. Exercise uses up energy, and energy comes from the glucose in your blood. Twenty years ago, doctors were reluctant to allow their patients with diabetes to participate in athletic activities.

Today, doctors and other health professionals are aware of the benefits of exercise. Not only does exercise help make you feel better by releasing endorphins, the so-called feel-good hormones, but regular exercise helps control your weight, tone your muscles, and control your insulin levels. Studies show that regular exercise not only helps prevent type 2 diabetes but may also help some people with type 2 diabetes avoid medication. The key to exercise is consistency balanced with diet. Vigorous exercise every now and then is likely to do more harm than good. You have to make a regular exercise schedule and stick to it. You also must remember to monitor your

If you take insulin, you must learn to recognize that different types of activities use up different calorie values. You need this information so that you can adjust your food intake accordingly. Excessive or extra exercise can leave you with too little blood glucose. You should be prepared for this by carrying a snack with you when you exercise. Test your blood sugar before you exercise; if it is low, you may have to raise it. If you participate in after-school sports and the coach calls for that extra practice, be prepared by bringing a fast sugar food with you. If you begin to experience the symptoms of low blood sugar, stop practicing and take care of yourself immediately. It is also a good idea to have a high-carbohydrate snack before you begin exercise.

Remember that exercise must be balanced with insulin. Exercise burns up extra glucose in the blood when there is a sufficient supply of insulin in the body. If insulin is not balanced with exercise, you may find your glucose levels rising after a workout. If you find that exercise raises your blood sugar levels, you may have to take more insulin or forgo that extra workout and wait until your glucose level falls. With a little practice, you will be able to find the right balance of exercise and insulin that will work for you.

You should try to perform some form of exercise at least three times a week. The most basic and simplest form of exercise is walking. Or you may want to join a gym. If you use insulin, you want to be sure to tell your doctor about the types of exercise you do, especially active sports such as football, cheerleading, or gymnastics. This way, he or she can make certain that additional calories are added to your diet to keep your glucose levels from dropping too low. Remember that your goal is to balance diet, exercise, and insulin. You cannot neglect any part of this balance if you want to control your diabetes.

BALANCING EXERCISE WITH DIABETES

glucose levels before and after exercise so that you may adjust your medication accordingly. Remember, too, that exercise alone will not do the trick. Exercise must be balanced with a healthy diet in order to be effective.

Before exercising, check your blood sugar level because exercise tends to lower it. If your blood sugar is low or some time has passed since your last meal, have a snack before exercising. There are also times when exercising will increase your blood sugar level. If your blood sugar level is over 300 mg/dl, you should either wait for the level to decrease or inject some insulin before exercising.

CHAPTER 9

This section focuses on the equipment you will need to use to monitor and control your diabetes. The different kinds and brands of equipment, how they work, how to maintain them, and what to look for when buying equipment are discussed.

Some lancets are used only for sight-reading; some can be read by machine and sight; and others can be read only by machine. Not all lancets fit all machines, so make sure if you have a machine that you are getting lancets that will fit it. Some machines are shaped like large markers. Others are shaped like powder compacts. Some lancet names are BD Micro-Fine Lancets, EasyStick, E-Zlets, Monoject, Soft Touch, Sugar System, Surelet, and Unilet-Lite. Some types of lancing machines are BD Autolance, Glucolet, Dialet, ExacTech, Monoject, Pen-It, and Soft Touch.

GLUCOSE MONITORS

Glucose monitors are small enough to carry in your pocket or purse. They weigh less than a pound, run on batteries, and take only a few minutes of your time. Like every kind of machine, you need to know how to operate it properly. The FDA reports that many users

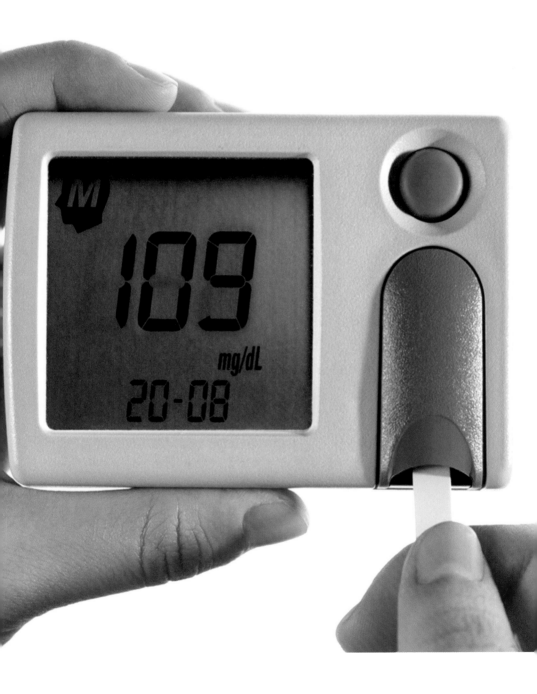

of glucose monitors use them incorrectly. In part, this is because many of the manufacturers' instructions are not very clear; also, the patients sometimes do not read the instructions carefully or do not consult a pharmacist or health care provider for assistance. Here is what you should do if you are using a glucose monitor:

1. Make sure you have it calibrated correctly. If your initial setting is incorrect, then all of your readings will be wrong as well. Some of the newer machines do not require calibration.
2. Read the manufacturer's instructions carefully. If you don't understand them, look for a toll-free number on the monitor's packaging or look online for additional information. Call the number to get in touch with someone who can walk you through the instructions.
3. Get professional instructions from your pharmacist, someone on your health care team, or someone who uses the same type of monitor successfully. Don't take chances and unnecessary risks by trying to do something you are not familiar with by yourself.
4. Always use fresh strips and supplies, and make certain you keep your meter clean.

Glucose monitors have taken a lot of the guesswork out of glucose testing. Some brands even come in different colors and styles to match your personal tastes.

What Should You Ask Before Buying a Glucose Monitor?

- What is the cost of the meter and the supplies? Glucose monitors vary in cost from about $50 to over $100. If the meter is relatively inexpensive but the supplies are twice as high as those for other meters, it will cost you more money in the long run.
- How easy is it to get supplies? If the manufacturer cannot keep up with demand, you will be left with a meter and no supplies. There are plenty of manufacturers of monitors, so comparison shop. Consult with your health care team for advice.
- How much blood does the meter require?
- Is the meter easy to clean?
- Is it easy to calibrate?
- Is it easy to read?
- What kind of data management is required? Do you write your own record, or do you need something more sophisticated?
- Can the meter detect interference that may be caused by other medications?
- Can you test it before you buy it?
- Does the manufacturer offer training in its use?
- What kind of warranty or guarantee does it have? Is there toll-free number you can call twenty-four hours a day? What kind of repair policies does the manufacturer have? Can you talk to people who use this meter?

GLYCOSYLATED HEMOGLOBIN TEST

The glycosylated hemoglobin test is called a long-term test. It is also known as the hemoglobin A1C test. This test is usually done every three to six months. It tests a blood sample to see how much sugar coating is on a red blood cell. Red blood cells live approximately 120 days, and the sugar in the blood coats the cells. The more sugar in the blood, the more sugar on the red blood cell. Because the life span of a red blood cell is only about four months, an analysis of the blood sample gives a fairly accurate description of what the blood sugar range was over several weeks. Glycosylation is the sugar coating process that goes on in the bloodstream. Ideally, the results will show a reading about the same as for someone without diabetes, if the diabetic is performing the right control measures.

INJECTING INSULIN

One of the basic ways to inject insulin into the body is by using a syringe. Some syringes can be used more than once, but only if the needle is straight, sharp, and sterile. Do not reuse a syringe if the needle is bent. Always sterilize the needle before you use it again. Most plastic syringes are designed to be thrown away after one use. Glass syringes are meant to be used again, but remember that these instruments must be kept sterile and cannot be left lying around where others have access to them. You can sterilize glass

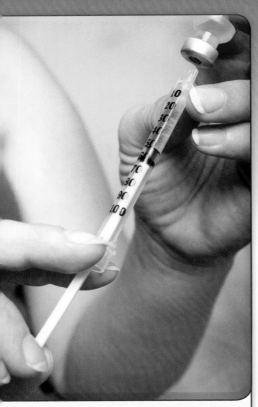

Syringes are a good way to administer insulin. They are simple to use and inexpensive. Talk to your doctor about finding the best injection technique for you.

syringes and nonplastic needles by boiling them.

Never use a syringe that is dirty. Never leave a used syringe lying around. Never simply throw a used syringe in the trash. Be considerate of others. Make certain that you wrap the needle carefully so others, especially the people who take away your trash, do not accidentally stick themselves with it.

Make sure the syringes you buy match the insulin strength and dosage you are injecting. In the United States, the most common is U-100 insulin (100 units), so you would buy a U-100 syringe. If your syringe holds less than your dose, you will not be getting enough insulin. Make certain you can read the numbers on the syringe. If the unit marks are too small or too close together, you may want to obtain a different syringe. Some syringes have plungers that are a different color so that you can read the marks more easily.

Compare prices and pharmacies. If you find a cheaper price at a pharmacy far from you, talk to the pharmacy nearest you. Usually they will match the price to keep your business. Keep an extra syringe on hand in case you break one.

Infusers

Some people use infusers to limit injections. With an infuser, a needle is placed under the skin and taped into place, and insulin is then injected into the needle rather than the skin. Infusers must be changed every two or three days.

Pens

The pen is a newer way to inject insulin. It uses cartridges just like an ink pen and usually costs less than $50. The pen is easy to carry and easy to use. Some are even disposable. You can carry an insulin pen right in your pocket.

The pen contains a needle and an insulin cartridge. When you are ready to give yourself an injection, you screw the needle onto the special end of the pen, make certain you have the correct dose (pens usually have a dial to adjust the dose), and then give yourself the injection. Not all forms of insulin are available in cartridge form. Right now lente and ultralente, the long-acting insulins, are not available for the pens.

Jet Injectors

The jet injector is a high-speed pen without a needle. The jet injector shoots insulin directly into you, under your skin. It is relatively painless and good for people who

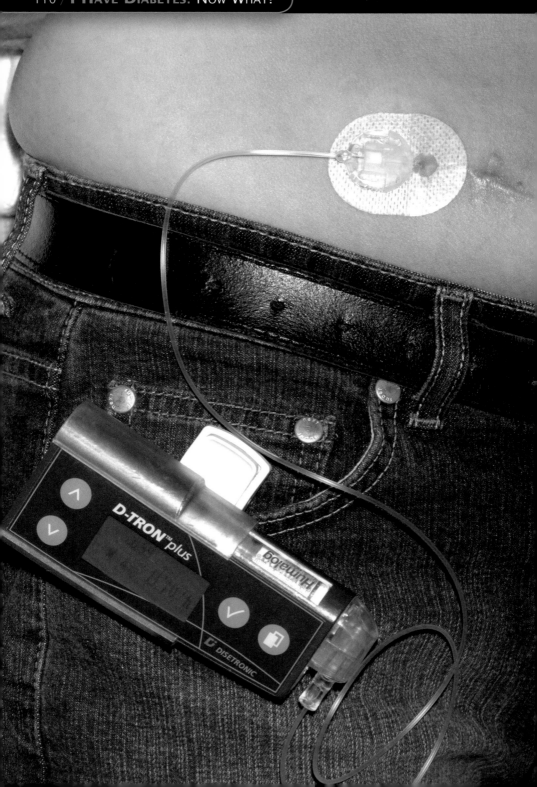

really hate needles. This is also a good insulin delivery system for those who have to take several shots a day. Jet injectors can get pretty expensive.

Pumps

Many people with type 1 diabetes are now using insulin pumps to deliver their insulin. Using a pump, which is an insulin infusion device, can greatly increase your freedom because, when used properly, it provides better control over your diabetes. Pumps are often recommended for people with brittle diabetes. Insulin pumps are also called open-loop systems. An insulin pump is about the size of a pager. It consists of a plastic case containing a large syringe called a pump reservoir, a battery-operated pump, and a computer chip. The pump reservoir holds the insulin, and the computer chip is programmed to deliver a certain amount of insulin. Plastic tubing runs from the pump to the delivery needle, also called a catheter needle. This is called the infusion set.

The needle is placed under your skin (subcutaneously), usually on the abdomen, but not where any clothing will interfere with it. Some people wear the pump hooked to a belt. Others wear it in a pocket. Women sometimes attach the pump to their bra. You wear the pump even when you sleep. The pump administers small doses of insulin all day long. The small doses of insulin are

Insulin pumps are probably the treatment that most closely resembles having a healthy pancreas. It delivers insulin twenty-four hours a day and offers more flexibility with food intake.

called the basal rate. The continuous delivery of insulin keeps the blood glucose levels within normal ranges all day long and through the night. This continuous delivery of insulin helps control the dawn phenomenon. The pump is programmed to give larger doses of insulin (a bolus dose) to balance out the amount of food eaten. Pumps are excellent for people who wish to maintain tight control over their diabetes. Because you control the insulin amount by simple programming, you can deliver different amounts of insulin without many injections. With a pump, you have only one injection every two or three days when you change the infusion set.

Most people who use pumps have found their lives less complicated. Nicole Johnson said she would not have been able to keep up her hectic schedule during her reign as Miss America if it had not been for her pump.

Although using a pump seems to make life easier for some people by allowing them to avoid several manual injections a day and by maintaining a steady dosage of insulin, that doesn't mean the pump relieves you of responsibility. In fact, while the pump means freedom from giving yourself injections, it also comes with a whole list of responsibilities.

Before You Buy a Pump

Other things to consider before you buy a pump:

- Since your pump runs on a computer chip, you need to make sure that the pump you are considering meets or exceeds electromagnetic interference immunity standards. This means that other electronic devices will not interfere with your pump.

- Make sure the pump you are considering has some sort of monitor that will alert you if insulin is not being delivered properly.
- Check to see if there is a safety range in the insulin delivery program so that you don't accidentally set the program for an unsafe dosage.
- Get information about different pumps. Compare costs and benefits. Find out what kind of technical support the manufacturer offers. Check all the warranties and guarantees that come with the pump you are considering. Buying a pump that has a limited warranty is not going to be extremely helpful if the pump motor isn't covered. Read the fine print. Ask others who use the pump.
- Pumps are expensive. Some can cost as much as $5,000. Don't assume that your insurance will cover the cost of one. Check first.
- If you have done all of your research and you are willing to assume all of the responsibilities that go with having a pump but your doctor is unwilling to go along, ask another member of your diabetes health care team to intervene. If your doctor is not an endocrinologist or a diabetologist, he or she may not be as familiar with the pump as someone who specializes in diabetes.

If you are considering using a pump, here are some things you need to be aware of:

- You must still decide with the advice of your health care provider how much insulin to program the pump to deliver.

- You must monitor the syringe that contains the insulin supply, the tubing, the battery, your skin, and your blood glucose levels. The major advantage of short-acting insulin is that it has a predictable absorption pattern, unlike NPH or ultralente. The major disadvantage is that there is no backup supply of insulin in your body if your pump fails. There is no emergency reservoir of insulin in your pump or in your body. When you're out, you're out. This puts you at risk for a quick slide into DKA (diabetic coma). Never begin a day without checking your reservoir and your blood glucose level. The syringe should be checked daily to ensure that you don't run out of insulin. Pumps use regular insulin, which is short-acting.

- You must change the infusion set every two or three days. This is an important responsibility.

- Most pumps come with an alarm that beeps if your battery is running low. If you hear this beep, don't wait until the last minute; replace the battery immediately. Know in advance how long a battery is supposed to last. Write the information down. Some pumps require that you send the battery back to the manufacturer for replacement. If that's the case with yours, make certain you have a spare. Make sure that the tubing remains clear and unbent. A kink in the tubing can impede the delivery of insulin. Make certain the needle is securely in place. And check your blood glucose levels often. Frequent testing ensures that you are aware of any problem before it becomes too big to handle.

- People who use the pumps are at risk for developing skin infections at the insertion site. So make certain you check it daily. And make sure you keep your skin clean.

Today, there are a lot of support groups in communities and on the Internet for people who pump.

CHAPTER 10

The teenage years are a time of experimentation. For someone with diabetes, there is no room for experimentation with anything that can alter your glucose levels or affect your health. You may be invited to a party where other kids are drinking or taking drugs. It's not always easy to "just say no," especially when you're with your friends or people you want to impress. But by saying yes to drugs or doing something that you know will affect your diabetes, you are endangering your health.

ALCOHOL

If you have diabetes, alcohol can be dangerous to you. Alcohol is full of calories. It has double the calories per gram that fat does. Beer and most mixed drinks contain carbohydrates. Drinking alcohol will initially raise your glucose levels. If you drink on an empty stomach your blood sugar could drop very quickly and you may go into a diabetic coma. This is because your liver cannot process alcohol and release glucose at the same time. Many diabetes medicines warn that mixing alcohol with the medicine could cause serious problems.

Another thing to remember is that a person experiencing hypoglycemia can appear to be drunk to others. Although the symptoms are different for hypoglycemia (low blood sugar) and for hyperglycemia (high blood sugar), your friends likely cannot tell the difference. If you are drinking at a party and go into DKA, your friends may just think you've had too much to drink and not recognize that you are sliding into hyperglycemia. If you have type 1 diabetes, you need to know that alcohol is poison to the nerves, and as a diabetic you are already at risk for potential nerve damage. Alcohol has been linked to the development of diabetic retinopathy. Alcohol is also harmful to the liver, heart, and kidneys.

So what should you do if you are at a party and alcohol is served? You should say you don't want any. You do not have to explain. If someone insists that you have a drink, remember the dangers to yourself. Would a friend insist that you put yourself in danger? Of course not. If you have to say no, say it. It won't be easy, but after a while, it gets easier.

DRUG USE

Drugs are dangerous for people without diabetes, and those with diabetes can face serious health consequences. Controlling your diabetes is vital for keeping yourself healthy. Drugs just get in the way of that goal.

- Cocaine raises blood pressure and blood glucose. Cocaine can cause irregular heartbeat and eventually heart disease.

- Diet pills increase heart rate and decrease appetite. This can result in low blood sugar and can increase the chances of hypoglycemia.
- Marijuana increases your appetite. It gives you the "munchies." If you break out of your dietary habits while you are on marijuana, your blood sugar will rise. Because marijuana can also cause lethargy, you may not care that your blood sugar is rising and may thus do nothing to alter it. The result could be DKA.
- Tranquilizers, muscle relaxants, and sleeping pills slow down your breathing and can hide the signs of hypoglycemia.

It is not easy to remember to monitor your blood glucose levels when you are high on drugs. Using drugs or alcohol when you have diabetes is irresponsible and is not a way to take control of your disease.

TOBACCO

You already know about the dangers of smoking for people without diabetes. For people with diabetes, the dangers are even greater.

Smoking narrows the blood vessels and decreases circulation to the limbs. More than 90 percent of diabetic limb amputations are on smokers. Smoking also increases the risks for diabetics of developing heart disease, kidney disease, nerve disease, and eye disease. These are diseases that diabetics are already at greater risk of developing than are people in the general population.

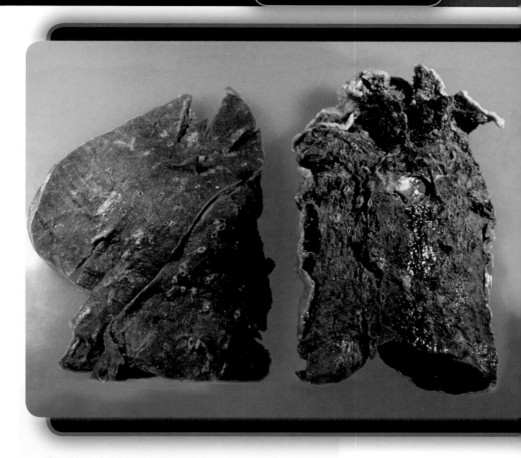

Smoking is dangerous whether or not you have diabetes. But the risks of disease increase with diabetes. Shown above are a healthy lung *(left)* and a smoker's lung *(right)*.

Nicotine, the additive ingredient in tobacco, contributes to heart disease. Tobacco smoke coats your lungs with residue that inhibits their ability to clean themselves. Weakened lungs make a person more susceptible to respiratory infections such as bronchitis. The carbon monoxide in cigarette smoke also cuts down on the oxygen supply to the body, making exercise more difficult. Smoking is addictive; there is no question about it. If you smoke, stop now. If you are thinking about smoking, think again. If you need help in quitting, talk to members of your health care team now.

TATTOOS AND PIERCINGS

Tattoos and body piercings are becoming increasingly popular with young people. Generally it is illegal to have your body pierced in any way or get a tattoo without parental permission if you are a minor. Some states have outlawed tattoo and body piercing parlors. Nevertheless, that doesn't stop people from having their bodies pierced or getting tattoos.

Tattooing is a process where pigment is injected under the skin to produce permanent designs. Some people falsely believe that the dye from a tattoo seeps into your kidneys. It doesn't. It stays under your skin. The major problem for anyone getting a tattoo is making certain that they are in a clean, antiseptic environment and that the tattoo artist is a skilled professional, not just somebody's friend. Recently, actress Pamela Anderson announced that she had contracted hepatitis C from using a dirty tattoo needle. Having diabetes means your immune system is not always as strong as someone who doesn't have diabetes, so if you insist on having a tattoo and have your parents' permission, make certain you go to a place that is certified as a healthy environment.

Make certain you keep the tattoo clean and continue to monitor your glucose levels closely.

Something else to remember about getting a tattoo is that it lasts a lifetime. Be really certain that you want to have that big image of a flag or someone's name plastered across your arm or back forever.

There are alternatives to permanent tattoos. There is an endless supply of temporary tattoos that you can just wash off. There are also the more traditional henna tattoos. People have been using henna tattoos for centuries. Henna is a natural substance that will dye the skin. All that is required is some henna oil, a brush, and a friend who is a good artist. There are also henna tattoo kits for sale with designs included. This effect usually lasts about three weeks and there is no skin scraping, no needle, and no risk of infection. And best of all, if you don't like it, you know it will be gone soon.

Body piercing is not the same as getting a tattoo. Body piercing involves creating a hole in your body somewhere and inserting jewelry. Many people have their ears pierced, and if you do, you know how long it took for your earlobes to heal. However, piercing in your earlobe is not the same as piercing in your tongue, lips, or genitals. This is very risky behavior for a person with diabetes. The risk of infection is very high for body piercing involving your mouth or genitals. The healing time is from several weeks to several months with a constant chance of a serious infection and secondary infection (infection in another area caused by the first infection). The American Dental Association has come out strongly against the practice of piercing anywhere in the mouth or lips because of the dangers involved. Having diabetes magnifies these dangers. If you are intent on having a part of your body pierced, please talk with your diabetes health care team first.

Fatty and High Sugar Foods

Because you are in a period of rapid growth, your body requires more food than an adult's. Your diet plan probably has several snacks scattered throughout the day. If you go out to eat with your friends on the weekend or after school, you can use some of your snack food requirements. Not all junk food is bad for you. Like everything else, the key word is moderation. You can eat a slice of pizza or a burger but avoid having a bacon cheeseburger with a side of fries or onion rings. Pick one or the other. You can drink diet soda. More fast food places now offer salads or salad bars than in the past. Don't feel that you have to stay away from your friends when they go out to eat. And, of course, you can always say no when you are offered something you don't want or know you shouldn't eat.

Being Prepared

First of all, you should always have some sort of fast sugar food with you. Put it in your pocket or in your purse.

Diabetes should not interfere with any travel. But you need to plan ahead. Make certain you have enough medication with you. Don't pack it in a suitcase that might get lost. Make certain you have a copy of any prescriptions you may need. Carry fast sugar food with you. Remember, if you cross time zones, you need to adjust your medication accordingly.

- If you are going to another country and have to have immunizations first, make certain you get them well enough in advance to allow any bad reactions to be alleviated. Know where the hospitals are in the foreign country. Know how to ask for a doctor. Know how to say that you have diabetes in the local language.
- If you do get the flu while traveling, call your doctor. Be careful what medications you take. Decongestants can raise blood pressure. Some cough syrups contain sugar and alcohol. Follow your sick-day guidelines. Being sick increases stress, so be sure to monitor your glucose levels carefully so that you can adjust your insulin levels.

DIABETES AND TRAVEL

If anyone gives you a hard time, explain your situation. It would be helpful if you had a medical alert bracelet or medallion. If someone still gives you a hard time, ask to see the manager. There is no need for you to carry such massive amounts of food that it is obvious. Keep a supply in your pocket or bag. More often than not, no one will question you about it. Make certain that your friends know to call an ambulance if something happens to you.

Diabetes in Males

Some complications caused by diabetes affect males more than females, so you need to be on the watch for symptoms.

One of these is called distal symmetrical polyneuropathy. This complication can cause sexual dysfunction or impotence, the inability to maintain an erection. You increase your risk of developing this complication if you smoke, drink alcoholic beverages, or cannot keep your glucose levels under control. There is a tendency to think that just having diabetes will prevent a man from having an erection and, consequently, a healthy sex life. That is simply not true. Although some men with diabetes become impotent, others do not. So far, scientists have not established a direct link between diabetes and impotence. But some of the complications that develop from out-of- control diabetes may result in sexual dysfunction.

Out-of-control diabetes can inhibit growth. And because you cannot always control your glucose levels during the teenage years as well as you might want to, make sure your doctor measures your height at each visit.

After puberty, your insulin requirements may drop, so you need to monitor your blood glucose levels carefully so that you don't end up injecting too much insulin.

Diabetes in Females

Diabetes presents some different challenges to females that you need to be aware of.

Menstruation

If your diabetes is not properly controlled, your first period may be delayed. This is called amenorrhea, and it can cause serious problems for you, not only now but throughout your life. It is imperative that you begin to control your diabetes now. Proper diet and exercise along with insulin therapy can help normalize your blood glucose levels. Your health care team may recommend low doses of estrogen if you are over age sixteen.

Menstruation can raise and lower your glucose levels. This is partly because your body is releasing anti-insulin hormones. Your body does not manufacture or use insulin the way someone without diabetes does, so you need to compensate for this. It is common for young women to have to keep increasing amounts of insulin at night during the week before their period. Also, women who suffer from premenstrual syndrome (PMS) may be more prone to hypoglycemia during the week before their period. It is always important to follow your glucose level testing schedules, but if you are prone to insulin fluctuations during the week before your period, testing your glucose levels often is very important. If your blood glucose levels tend to rise during this time, there are some things you can do:

1. Consult your health care provider about increasing your insulin dose during this week.
2. Watch your diet and avoid extra carbohydrates.
3. Exercise more.

4. Monitor your blood glucose levels.

If your blood glucose levels fall during this time, try the following:

1. Consult your health care provider about decreasing your insulin dose during this week.
2. Watch your diet and take extra carbohydrates.
3. Exercise a little less during this time.
4. Monitor your blood glucose levels.

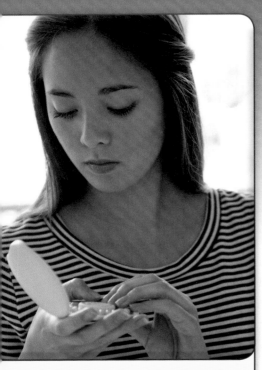

Like any medication, oral contraceptives may cause problems for diabetes sufferers. If you take birth control pills, talk to your doctor about possible adjustments to your medication.

Women have to be watchful for yeast infections. The signs of a yeast infection are vaginal itching and a white discharge. Yeast infections are caused by a fungus, *Candida albicans*, which flourishes on high blood glucose and moisture. Wear cotton underwear to decrease moisture. Sometimes you might develop a rash under your breasts. Your health care team can also recommend various powders and creams that will help keep rashes and yeast infections under control. As always, the first line of defense is to keep your diabetes under control as much as you can.

Birth Control

Not all oral contraceptives are good for women with diabetes. Some may increase your blood pressure. Some may make you gain weight. Some may increase your blood sugar level. Be careful about what you take, and always talk to your doctor about the side effects of any medications.

TYPE 2 DIABETES AND WEIGHT LOSS

If you are overweight and have been diagnosed with type 2 diabetes, your doctor has probably told you to lose weight. You need to monitor carefully your calorie and fat intake and develop a good exercise program. Ask a member of your health care team to help you develop an exercise plan you can stick to. There is a difference between being slightly overweight and being obese. If your doctor has diagnosed you as being obese, you face other health risks in addition to type 2 diabetes. Work with your diabetes educator to come up with a diet plan you and your family can live with. Absolutely stay away from fast food and nondiet sodas. Fast food is usually high in carbohydrates and nondiet sodas are high in empty calories.

Also remember this is your greatest growth period, and out-of-control diabetes can inhibit growth, not weight gain. In addition to working to control your diabetes, make sure your doctor measures your height at each visit.

Potential Eating Disorders

Because people with diabetes have to balance their food intake carefully, being too thin is not an option. Unfortunately, young women sometimes have such poor self-images that they avoid eating (anorexia) or they eat and then vomit (bulimia). These eating disorders can make you very sick and may even cause death. Withholding insulin (also called insulin purging) is another related disorder specific to people with diabetes. By withholding insulin, a young woman immediately increases her susceptibility to depression, which goes hand in hand with low self-esteem. She also places herself at risk of long-term disability or dying young. If having diabetes has affected your self-image to the point of withholding insulin, talk to your parents and a trained therapist. You need support NOW. Don't think you can handle this by yourself.

TAKING PRECAUTIONS DURING AN ILLNESS

When you are sick with the flu, a cold, or anything else, it's very easy to let your daily routine slide by. Don't! When you're sick, you must be very careful about maintaining your balance. Remember that in order for the body to repair itself quickly, it must have a steady supply of insulin. People who have diabetes do not have a steady supply of insulin and are at risk of developing more complications from any illness if they do not maintain a good insulin balance.

Always have your doctor's phone number close at hand. Let your doctor know that you are sick so that he or she can give you specific advice and medications.

If you take insulin, you must continue to take it just as you do every day. Not taking insulin when you are sick can cause serious complications and may bring on DKA. Your doctor may advise you to take extra insulin on those days that you are sick.

- Test your blood glucose levels at least four times a day.
- If you take insulin, test your urine for ketones at least twice a day.
- You need to eat the proper amount of food to balance your insulin intake. If you have difficulty keeping food down, take liquids, small sips at a time. Make certain the liquids contain carbohydrates if you are not eating.
- Drink plenty of fluids to prevent dehydration, especially if you have a fever. Write down how much you drink.
- Be careful of the medications you take. Aspirin can lower glucose levels. Check the labels for sugar and alcohol content.
- Get plenty of rest.

Make sure your teacher knows why you are out, and make arrangements to have a friend pick up any schoolwork and books that you will need to catch up on. Call your doctor (or go to the hospital if you cannot reach your doctor) if:

- Your blood glucose is greater than 225 mg/dl and your urine tests positive for ketones.
- You are vomiting and/or have diarrhea and you cannot take fluids.

You can decrease your chances of getting the flu by getting a flu shot every year. The Centers for Disease Control and Prevention (CDC) estimates that only about 40 percent of adult diabetics receive flu shots and that this percentage decreases considerably for younger people. Doctors at the CDC say that the failure to get a flu shot each fall causes thousands of people with diabetes to die from complications of the flu. Having the flu is not the same as having a cold. The flu is a viral respiratory infection that can lead to pneumonia. The flu can be very dangerous even for people who do not have diabetes, but it is especially so for those who do have chronic diseases such as diabetes. Remember, high blood glucose levels impair the body's ability to fight infection.

CHAPTER 11

You will have not one doctor but several because diabetes is a syndrome (a collection of several diseases). First you probably have a pediatrician, then an endocrinologist to check hormone levels and advise you and your family on various diabetes treatments. You should also have a diabetes educator to assist you in learning about the disease and to help you understand it better. A diabetes educator is the person to turn to with all sorts of questions you may have. A podiatrist will help you care for your feet, and an ophthalmologist or a retinologist will care for your eyes. You will probably have other health care professionals as well, such as a dietitian to help you plan a workable diet for your lifestyle, a psychologist to help you and other family members deal with the emotional stresses of diabetes, and a social worker to assist you and your family in finding community support programs as well as financial resources to pay for your treatment.

According to the ADA, these are things you should expect your health care team to ask about each time you meet:

1. Your blood glucose records. This information is important because your insulin may have to be adjusted at different times

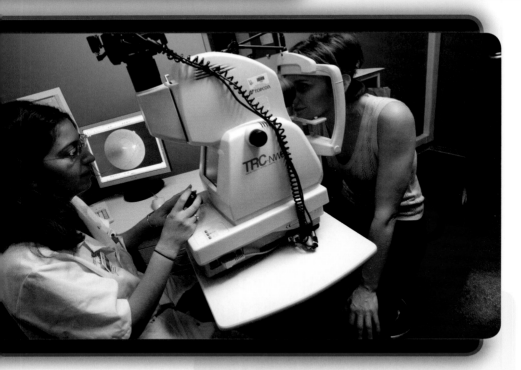

High glucose and high blood pressure from diabetes can damage the retina, vitreous fluid, lens, and optic nerve. Therefore, an ophthalmologist is an important member of your medical team.

throughout the day to compensate for different glucose levels.

2. Any life changes. Remember, stress affects diabetes.

3. If you've made any changes in your care program or if you've had any problems with it.

4. If you've been sick since your last visit. Remember that illness can affect your insulin level and that some illnesses may be related to your diabetes.

5. What medications you are on. Different medications can interact with each other and with insulin. If your

health care team has all of this knowledge, they can then make recommendations and substitutions as necessary to prevent complications.

6. Your menstrual periods, if you are a female.

If these questions aren't being asked, volunteer the information. If no one seems interested, then it may be time to look for a different health care team.

The following are things you should expect your health care team to do each time you meet:

1. Take blood for a glycohemoglobin test.
2. Take a urine sample.
3. Check your eyes.
4. Check your feet.
5. Check your weight.
6. Check your height.
7. Check your blood pressure.

If these things aren't being done, ask why not. If no one seems interested, then it may be time to look for a different health care team. There are other things you have a right to expect from your health care providers.

YOU HAVE A RIGHT TO BE TREATED WITH DIGNITY AND RESPECT

Sometimes older people tend to view teenagers as irresponsible and incapable of making good decisions. If any member of your health care team treats you with disrespect or doesn't clearly explain things, speak up. If you are unwilling to confront that person, tell another member of your health care team about it. Don't keep quiet and just worry about each visit with that person. That is just unnecessary stress.

Your doctor and each member of your health care team should talk with you about diabetes and your care. They should not lecture you. After all, it is supposed to be a team effort, and you are the most important member of the team. Don't forget that.

YOU HAVE A RIGHT TO ASK QUESTIONS AND EXPECT ANSWERS

Because you are not yet considered an adult, you may find that some members of your team are reluctant to discuss things about your disease with you. If you find that happening, you will have to become more assertive when you deal with those members of your team. If you are controlling your diabetes in a responsible manner, there is no reason why your health care team should not discuss all aspects of your treatment with you as well as your parents.

Speak up if you are not being informed. Or ask your parents not to accompany you into the doctor's office. Be prepared when you go to the doctor. Have a list of questions written down. Check them off as the doctor answers them for you.

YOU HAVE A RIGHT TO HAVE ALL PROCEDURES, TESTS, AND MEDICINES EXPLAINED TO YOU IN LANGUAGE THAT YOU, NOT JUST YOUR PARENTS, UNDERSTAND

If your doctor is not explaining things to you so that you understand them, he or she is doing you a disservice. After all, you are the one who has diabetes, and you are the one who is mostly responsible for controlling it. If your doctor uses words that you don't understand, interrupt and say, "I don't understand. Could you please explain it to me in other words?" Don't worry that you may sound as if you don't know what the doctor is talking about—you don't, and you need to.

YOU HAVE A RIGHT TO INFORMATION ABOUT THE VARIETY OF TREATMENTS AVAILABLE

Some doctors are partial to certain kinds of treatment and not to others. That does not give your doctor or any other member of your health care team the right to withhold any information about different kinds of available treatment. If you have heard about a new treatment, you have a right to expect your doctor to discuss the good and bad things about it.

If, after discussing a new treatment or procedure thoroughly, you and your parents decide to go ahead with it, you have a right to expect that your doctor and other members of your health care team will be supportive of your decision.

YOU HAVE A RIGHT TO PRIVACY

There may be some things you want to talk to your doctor or other members of your health care team about that you don't want your parents to know about. You may have questions about birth control, drugs, or how diabetes may affect your sex life in the future. Ask your doctor if he or she will maintain your confidence and not discuss your questions with your parents.

Don't assume that confidentiality is the rule. You are still considered a minor and under your parents' protection. If your confidentiality cannot be guaranteed, then you need to find someone else with whom you can discuss these matters. You may want to try a diabetes hotline or Web site or contact the American Diabetes Association for more information about sensitive topics.

If you find that you and your health care team don't get along for any of the reasons above or because your personalities just don't fit together, ask your parents about finding another doctor. It is important to get along with your health care team. You must feel comfortable when you are with any one of them. You must be able to trust their judgments and opinions. If you are not comfortable, you will always wonder if you are getting good advice.

YOUR HEALTH CARE TEAM AND YOU

Just as you have a right to expect certain things from your health care team, they have a right to expect certain things from you.

They have a right to expect you to be honest about your testing habits and record keeping. If you are only testing once or twice a day, don't tell anyone you are testing four or five times a day. You test in order to adjust your insulin dosage to your needs. If you are only testing once or twice a day, you are not adjusting according to your needs and you are not displaying a true record of your overall glucose levels.

Your doctor has a right to expect you to be honest about your eating habits and exercise. If you do not tell your doctor the truth about what you eat or how you exercise, he or she may make incorrect assumptions about your insulin adjustments. If you are reluctant to tell the truth because you don't want to seem irresponsible or you don't want your doctor to be angry, you are merely putting yourself at risk. First of all, if you do not follow your diet and exercise plan, you are not hurting your doctor, so he or she has no right to get angry. Second of all, if you are consistently breaking your diet and exercise rules, it may be that those particular rules are not good for you and your doctor may need to help you adjust them. However, if you are given several different plans and are unable to stick with any of them, maybe you need to ask yourself if you are being responsible or not.

You should be keeping a record of your glucose testing results. This should include the date and time of the testing and the results. You might also want to include any changes in your usual schedule that might have had an effect on your glucose level. You could draw a simple chart like this:

Day	Time	Results	Unusual Events

Or you may be able to get a free booklet from your health care team. There are also many software programs available on the Internet that you could use. Diabetes Research (http://www.diabetesresearch.com/) offers free online software for glucose monitoring. You can store all your information right on the Internet. The Diabetic Gourmet (http://www.diabeticgourmet. com/) has a variety of freeware that you can download on your computer and use. Find other free software by going to any search engine and typing "diabetes freeware." Or type "diabetes software" if you are interested in purchasing a program.

No matter what method you use, record keeping may help you normalize your schedule. You will be able to see at what times of the day your blood sugar is too high or too low and be able to make adjustments to help you maintain the proper balance.

Your health care team needs accurate information in order to help you. If you are not keeping records of your testing and insulin dosages, don't make excuses. Chances are they have already heard the same excuse from someone else. Keeping good records helps your health care team understand how your body is working, but more important, keeping good records lets you know how your body is working and is one of the steps toward tight control.

CHAPTER 12

THE FUTURE of DIABETES

Because diabetes is a chronic disease that so far has no known cure, the way diabetes affects your future depends very much on what you do to take care of yourself today. But there is some general information that you as a diabetic need to know about the world we live in. Although diabetes cannot be cured, it can be controlled, and because of this, there are very few limitations for you.

Federal law does prohibit people with insulin-dependent diabetes from serving in the armed forces, holding jobs as pilots, or holding jobs that require driving interstate vehicles. States or cities may have similar restrictions, but for the most part employers are urged to take each person as an individual. These laws are being challenged by many people as a result of the Americans with Disabilities Act of 1992. Since 1992, more than one thousand cases of job discrimination have been filed by people with diabetes. A few years ago, Ken Drugger, who has type 1 diabetes, successfully sued the Bureau of Alcohol, Tobacco and Firearms, forcing it to reconsider its policy of not allowing people with insulin-dependent diabetes to become criminal investigators or special agents. It took Drugger seven years to obtain his victory, but it is a victory for everyone with diabetes. In addition, the Americans with Disabilities Act

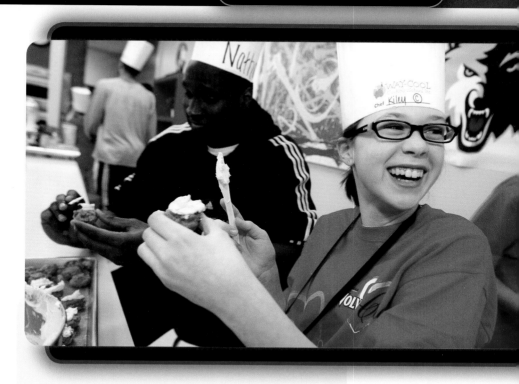

This January 2010 event, Way Cool Cooking School, gave college students a chance to teach kids with diabetes how to cook more diabetic friendly meals.

is working to revoke the ban against allowing people with diabetes to obtain commercial driver's licenses and pilot's licenses. You are not required to tell an employer that you have diabetes.

Having a Family

Diabetes should not prevent you from getting married and having children. If you are a woman with diabetes, you will need to practice tight control in order to

SLOWING THE OBESITY EPIDEMIC AND THE SURGE OF DIABETES

In the last several years, with obesity on the rise, many scientists and doctors are noticing that type 2 diabetes is on the rise as well. And it's striking people at younger ages.

Type 2 diabetes was once referred to as adult onset diabetes since it appeared mostly in people over the age of forty. But according to recent findings, around two million people between the ages of twelve and nineteen have "prediabetes," which are high glucose levels that could eventually turn into type 2 diabetes if left untreated.

So, what can people do to prevent diabetes?

- Boycott fast-food chains. Fast food is high in fat and sugar. A demand for better ingredients and healthier options could help drive fast-food chains to comply with healthier standards.
- Join or help organize a walk or fund-raiser for diabetes awareness.
- Talk to your principal or other school official about using fresh, local produce in school lunches.
- Make healthy food choices for yourself, even if you are not at risk for diabetes. People around you may take notice and make better choices for themselves.
- If you are at risk for diabetes, talk to your parents or family doctor about what you can do to avoid getting diabetes.
- If you have diabetes, help educate others about your disease.

maintain acceptable blood sugar levels when you are pregnant. You will probably see your doctor more than a pregnant woman without diabetes would. However, having diabetes should never stand in the way of leading a full and productive life.

ADVANCES IN TECHNOLOGY

Researchers are working on several types of noninvasive glucose monitors. One device under study uses near-infrared light that passes through the finger and "takes a picture" of what it sees, including the glucose in the blood. Another type of monitor being worked on is a skin patch that could extract glucose through the skin. Research is also being done on an implanted monitor that would monitor glucose levels all day long.

ADVANCES IN INSULIN DELIVERY

Researchers seem to be on the verge of developing a way to overcome the problems of taking insulin orally. Scientists have developed a small "bead" of protective material that would surround the insulin and prevent a person's digestive juices from destroying it. This would eliminate the need for injections for many people.

TRANSPLANTS

Scientists at the University of Massachusetts are working on a method to transplant islet cells from a healthy

Donor's cells for diabetic

For the first time, a living volunteer donor has been used to provide insulin-making pancreas cells to reverse a patient's diabetes; the donor cells were transplanted into the diabetic patient's liver.

Pancreas cells taken from donor

About half of donor's pancreas is removed

Insulin-making islet cells are extracted from donated pancreas tissue and purified

Pancreas islet cells

Make insulin, a hormone that helps body use glucose

Diabetic's pancreas does not make enough insulin or does not use it

Liver
Regulates chemical levels in blood, prepares fats for digestion

Pancreas
Makes insulin and enzymes that help body digest and use food

Islet cells injected

Islet cells from donor are injected through portal vein into patient's liver

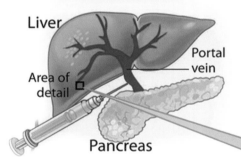

Liver

Area of detail

Portal vein

Pancreas

Implanted islet cells lodge in veins in liver; are sustained by blood vessels and tissue that grow around them

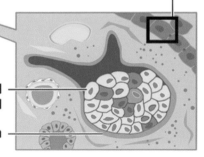

Liver cells

Implanted islet cell

Vein

Source: National Diabetes Information Clearinghouse, Dr. Jose Oberholzer of the University of Illinois at Chicago
Graphic: Chicago Tribune

© 2005 KRT

pancreas to a diabetic person's pancreas. Canadian researchers are working on the same type of program. These transplants are important because they would enable the body of a person with diabetes to produce normal levels of insulin on its own.

PREVENTIVE MEASURES

The National Institute of Diabetes and Digestive and Kidney Diseases (NIDDKD) is doing a study to see if insulin therapy undertaken before the onset of type 1 diabetes can prevent the condition from developing in those who test positive in tests such as the islet cell antibody test.

The process of transplanting pancreas cells into a diabetic patient's liver was first reported in a 2000 issue of the *New England Journal of Medicine*.

CHAPTER 13

HOW TO BE PREPARED

All the things you need to do to control your diabetes may seem pretty overwhelming, especially if you have just been diagnosed. It is true that diabetes can affect every aspect of your life, but diabetes does not have to control your life if you are willing to control your diabetes. Sometimes it is hard enough just being a teenager without having the complications of diabetes.

Remember, you did nothing to get diabetes. It is not caused by eating candy bars. Scientists do not yet know why some people get diabetes and others don't. Having diabetes means that you need to control your balance of insulin and glucose in order to prevent hypoglycemia and hyperglycemia and to avoid or delay future complications. You do this through diet, exercise, and sometimes medication or insulin, depending on the type of diabetes you have. Just because you don't take insulin doesn't mean your diabetes isn't serious. All diabetes is serious and potentially life threatening. There are some basic things to do if you have diabetes:

- Monitor your glucose levels regularly and keep an accurate log of those readings.
- Get into a routine of checking your body for scratches, cuts, or sores.
- Practice good oral and body hygiene.

- Eat a healthy diet with plenty of fruits, vegetables, and fiber.
- Read the labels on food to find out the ingredients.
- Exercise regularly.
- If you take insulin, make certain you follow your doctor's instructions and be sure you are always prepared with an emergency insulin kit.
- See your dentist regularly.
- Have yearly eye exams.
- Get a flu shot each fall.
- If you get sick, call your doctor.
- Give yourself a pat on the back now and then for a job well done.

There are some basic things not to do if you have diabetes:

- Don't smoke.
- Don't use alcohol or recreational drugs.
- Don't wear tight clothing, especially on your legs and feet.
- Don't stop taking insulin or any other medication unless your doctor tells you to stop.
- Don't try to fix ingrown toenails yourself.

Follow these tips to better prepare yourself for coping with diabetes:

- Always keep extra supplies of insulin or oral medications handy for emergencies. Know the type of

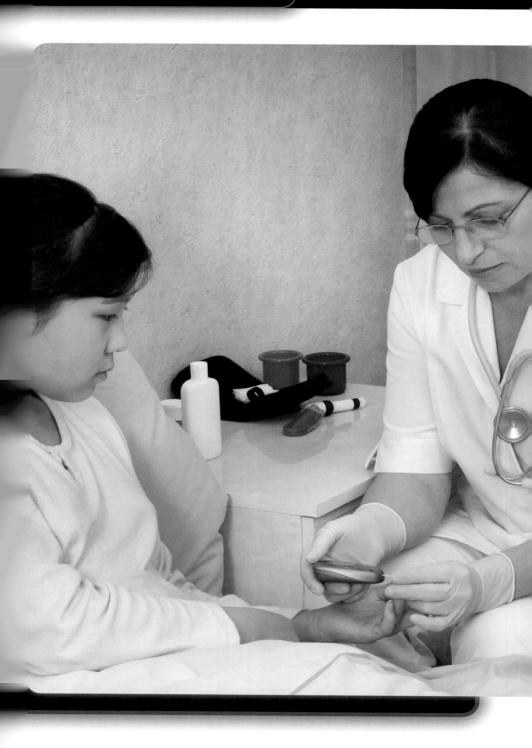

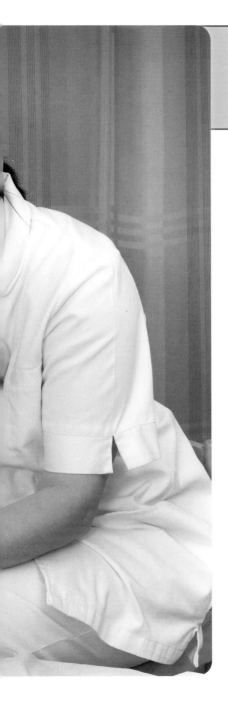

Always have your doctor's phone number close by. Program it into your cell phone, or write it down in a place where it can easily be found.

medication or insulin you take and how much.

- Have your doctor's phone number with you all the time. Know how to reach him or her on weekends, at night, or on holidays.

- Have a plan for sick days before you get sick. Follow the sick day guidelines and the advice of your doctor.

- Because fluctuating levels of glucose are the most common cause of complications for people with diabetes, it is a good idea to review how to manage them.

- Frequent testing will usually let you know if your glucose levels need to be treated with insulin, exercise, or food. Keeping good records will help you see if there is a

pattern to your glucose levels so that you can antici-
pate complications before they occur.

- You need to make the people around you aware of
the differences between hypoglycemia and hyperglycemia and what to do to treat either one of them.

- It is important to understand that the better you control your diabetes, the less chance you have of
developing complications related to diabetes.

Remember, you are not alone. You have your health
care team for your medical needs. You have friends and
family for your emotional needs. And there are millions
of people with diabetes throughout the world. Some of
them live in your own neighborhood. Meet them and
share your experiences and learn from theirs. Don't let
diabetes control your life. Make it your job to control
your diabetes.

Good luck!

1. How do I know when I need to call my doctor or go to an emergency room?

2. Should I get a pump?

3. Whom can I talk to about my diabetes?

4. How do I know how different foods will affect my blood sugar level?

5. Whom do I need to tell that I have diabetes? What should I tell my friends?

6. Can I still play sports?

7. Will I be able to have children? Will they have diabetes, too?

8. Why do my blood sugar levels get funky some days even though I'm being careful?

9. Can I drive? How do I know what activities I can participate in safely?

10. What should I carry with me for emergencies?

MYTH

Diabetes is caused by eating too much sugar, and people with diabetes shouldn't eat sugar.

FACT

Diabetes is caused by too little insulin, not by eating too much sugar. Sugar is just one of the carbohydrates people with diabetes must keep track of. For people with type 2 diabetes, sugar by itself isn't the key issue—their whole way of eating may be, though. If the body is having trouble using insulin, then keeping track of carbohydrates and calories is important.

MYTH

If type 2 diabetes isn't causing any problems, then it can be ignored until it acts up.

FACT

Undiagnosed or ignored type 2 diabetes causes major health and quality of life problems. It's incredibly hard to realize that something that isn't bothering you is really hurting you. It's also hard to realize that seemingly harmless behavior like not getting exercise, drinking soft drinks, and eating fast-food burgers can be harmful to your health. Diabetes complications take some time to develop, but the more aware a person is of his or her habits, the better his or her health is likely to be.

MYTH

Vanilla, cinnamon, aloe juice, chromium, or vitamin supplements can be used to control diabetes.

FACT

Juices and supplements have not yet been proved to control diabetes, though herbs and minerals are being studied as possibilities for controlling diabetes. If you hear about an alternative therapy that sounds interesting or that someone tells you is getting results, talk to your health team about it first. Supplements can interact badly with your medicines.

MYTH

Diabetes is contagious.

FACT

You didn't catch diabetes from somebody, and no one can catch it from you. If someone in your family (a blood relative) has diabetes, there is a greater chance of you getting it. That's not because you caught it, but because a vulnerability to the disease can be inherited.

MYTH

If you have diabetes, it's your fault because you have an unhealthy diet.

FACT

Both types 1 and 2 diabetes are caused by a genetic disposition. We don't know what sparks type 1 diabetes in someone with type 1 genes, but in type 2, poor diet, lack of exercise, and being overweight increase your chances of getting it.

SHARE YOUR STORY

Teen Health & Wellness: Real Life, Real Answers (*teenhealthandwellness.com*) offers teens an opportunity to share their personal stories for online publication.

Sharing stories is a powerful way to connect with other people. By telling your story, you can reach out and help someone better understand his or her own experience. If your story is accepted for publication, you can take pride in being published online as part of an award-winning database. You will also receive a letter of commendation and monetary gift. For more information about the Personal Story Project, go to *teenhealthandwellness.com/static/personalstoryproject*.

Teen Health & Wellness: Real Life, Real Answers is a database designed for teens on issues relating to health, fitness, alcohol, drugs, mental health, family life, and much more. Check your school or local library for access.

ABOUT DR. JAN

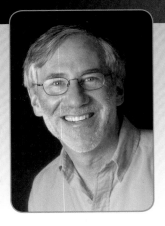

Dr. Jan Hittelman is a licensed psychologist with over twenty years of experience working with teens, children, adults, and families in a variety of settings.

In addition to clinical practices in California, Colorado, and New York, he has specialized in program development in partnership with school systems, psychiatric hospitals, correctional facilities and the courts, outpatient settings, residential treatment facilities, and private nonprofit organizations.

He founded Compass House, a nonprofit counseling collaborative for teens and their families. He launched Boulder Psychological Services in 2007.

Dr. Hittelman also authors a monthly newspaper column entitled "Surviving the Teenage Years" in the *Boulder Daily Camera*, writes monthly columns for the Boulder Valley School District under the sponsorship of the Parent Engagement Network, and publishes an online question-and-answer column for teens in the Rosen Publishing Group's online resource Teen Health & Wellness.

Teen Health & Wellness: Real Life, Real Answers (*http://www.teenhealthandwellness.com*) is a database designed for teens on issues relating to health, fitness, alcohol, drugs, mental health, family life, and much more. Check your school or local library for access.

GLOSSARY

basal dose A low, continual dose of insulin given by an insulin pump.

blood sugar Also known as blood glucose, it's the amount of sugar found in the bloodstream.

bolus dose A large dose of insulin taken before meals or snacks.

dawn phenomenon A high blood sugar count (hyperglycemia) upon waking up in the morning.

diabetes mellitus Medical term for diabetes.

dialysis The process of removing impure blood from a patient through a vein, cleaning it, and returning it through a vein.

DKA (diabetic ketoacidosis) A high amount of glucose in the blood that can lead to a diabetic coma.

endocrinologist A doctor who specializes in the glands of the body that manufacture hormones.

endorphins Hormones released by the body that make a person feel good.

finger stick Method of obtaining a drop of blood to test for glucose.

glaucoma Eye disease marked by increasing pressure within the eyeball that can result in loss of vision.

glucose A simple sugar that the body converts from food to provide energy to the body.

hyperglycemia Too much sugar in the bloodstream.

hypoglycemia Low amount of sugar in the bloodstream.

insulin Hormone produced by the pancreas that helps
move glucose from the bloodstream into the cells
where it can be used for energy.

insulin resistance Ineffective use of insulin by the body.

ketones The waste product of the body's breaking
down fats to use for energy.

pancreas The organ behind the stomach responsible
for producing insulin and glucagon.

podiatrist A doctor who specializes in caring for the feet.

retinologist A doctor who specializes in caring for the
eyes, especially the retina.

SMBG (self-monitoring of blood glucose) Daily testing
of the glucose levels in the blood, often through the
use of a finger stick and a blood glucose monitor.

FOR MORE INFORMATION

American Association of Diabetes Educators
100 West Monroe, Suite 400
Chicago, IL 60603
(312) 644-2233
(800) 338-3633
(800) TEAMUP (for referral to a diabetes educator in
    your area)
Web site: http://www.aadenet.org

An association of healthcare professionals dedicated to promoting self-management as the way to help diabetes patients help themselves.

American Diabetes Association (ADA)
National Office
1701 North Beauregard Street
Alexandria, VA 22311
(800) 232-3472
Web site: http://www.diabetes.org

Association with the primary goal of helping to prevent and cure diabetes and to improve the lives of people affected by it.

American Dietetic Association
216 West Jackson Boulevard
Chicago, IL 60606-6995
(800) 877-1600
(312) 899-0040
Web site: http://www.eatright.org

The world's largest organization of food and nutrition professionals, dedicated to providing up-to-date information on food and nutrition.

Canadian Diabetes Association

15 Toronto Street, Suite 800

Toronto, ON M5C2E3

Canada

(800) 226-8464

Web site: http://www.diabetes.ca/Section_Main/
  contact.asp

Canadian association with the primary goal of helping to prevent and cure diabetes and to improve the lives of people affected by it.

Diabetes Exercise and Sports Association (DESA)

P.O. Box 1935

Litchfield Park, AZ 85340

(800) 898-IDAA (898-4322)

Web site: http://www.diabetes-exercise.org

An organization with the goal of enhancing the quality of life for diabetes patients through fitness and exercise.

Juvenile Diabetes Research Foundation (Canada)

7100 Woodbine Avenue, Suite 311

Markham, ON L3R 5J2

Canada

(905) 944-8700

Web site: http://www.jdfc.ca/index_english.html

Foundation dedicated to research and an increased understanding of Type 1 diabetes

Juvenile Diabetes Research Foundation International

120 Wall Street
New York, NY 10005
(800) JDF-CURE (533-2873)
(212) 785-9500
E-mail: info@jdfcure.org
Web site: http://www.jdrf.org

Foundation dedicated to research and an increased understanding of Type 1 diabetes.

National Institute of Diabetes and Digestive and Kidney Diseases (NIDDKD)

Building 31, Room 9A04
Center Drive, MSC 2560
Bethesda, MD 20892-2560
(301) 496-3583
Web site: http://www.niddk.nih.gov

National institute that conducts and supports basic and clinical research for diabetes and digestive and kidney diseases.

Weight Control Information Network

1 WIN Way
Bethesda, MD 20892-3665
(800) WIN-8098 (946-8098)
(301) 984-7378
E-mail: win@info.niddk.nih.gov

Web site: http://www.niddk.nih.gov/health/nutrit/
   win.htm

*An information service dedicated to providing information on exercise,
nutrition, and weight control to the general public.*

WEB SITES

Due to the changing nature of Internet links, Rosen
Publishing has developed an online list of Web sites
related to the subject of this book. This site is updated
regularly. Please use this link to access the list:

http://www.rosenlinks.com/411/dia

FOR FURTHER READING

American Diabetes Association. *American Diabetes Association Complete Guide to Diabetes*. New York, NY: Bantam, 2006.

Bernstein, Richard K. *Dr. Bernstein's Diabetes Solution: The Complete Guide to Achieving Normal Blood Sugars*. New York, NY: Little, Brown, 2007.

Bliss, Michael. *The Discovery of Insulin*. Chicago, IL: University of Chicago Press, 2007.

Brand-Miller, Jennie, M.D., Kaye Foster-Powell, Stephen Colaguiri, M.D., and Alan Barclay. *The New Glucose Revolution for Diabetes: The Definitive Guide to Managing Diabetes and Prediabetes Using the Glycemic Index*. Cambridge, MA: Da Capo Press, 2007.

Brand-Miller, Jennie, M.D., Kaye Foster-Powell, and David Mendosa. *The New Glucose Revolution: What Makes My Blood Glucose Go Up . . . and Down?: 101 Frequently Asked Questions About Your Blood Glucose Levels*. Cambridge, MA: Da Capo Press, 2006.

Colberg, Sheri R. *Diabetic Athlete's Handbook*. Champaign, IL: Human Kinetics Publishers, 2008.

Colberg, Sheri R., and Steven V. Edelman. *50 Secrets of the Longest Living People with Diabetes*. Cambridge, MA: Da Capo Press, 2007.

Conkling, Winifred, and Deborah Mitchell. *Living Well with Diabetes*. New York, NY: St. Martin's, 2009.

Fox, Charles, and Anne Kilvert. *Type 1 Diabetes: Answers at Your Fingertips*. 6th ed. London, England: Class Publishing, 2007.

Hanas, Ragnar, M.D. *Type 1 Diabetes: A Guide for Children, Adolescents, Young Adults—and Their Caregivers*. Cambridge, MA: Da Capo Press, 2005.

Masharani, Umesh. *Diabetes Demystified: A Self-Teaching Guide*. New York, NY: McGraw-Hill, 2007.

Mayo Clinic. *The Essential Diabetes Book*. New York, NY: Time, 2009.

Reddy, Sethu. *The Cleveland Clinic Guide to Diabetes*. New York, NY: Kaplan, 2009.

Rubin, Alan L., M.D. *Type 1 Diabetes for Dummies*. Hoboken, NJ: Wiley, 2008.

Smith, Tom. *Living with Type 1 Diabetes*. London, England: Sheldon Press, 2009.

Weiss, Michael A., and Martha Mitchell Funnell. *The Little Diabetes Book You Need to Read*. Philadelphia, PA: Running Press, 2007.

INDEX

A

acarbose, 88
adult-onset diabetes, 14
alcohol consumption, 64,
116–117, 118, 124, 147
alpha-glucosidase inhibi-
tors, 88
Americans with Disabilities
Act of 1992, 140–141
amputations, 68, 118
Anderson, Pamela, 120
anorexia, 128
antibiotics, 69
Aretaeus, 8
athletics and diabetes,
49–50, 54–56, 57, 74,
87, 100, 101, 151

B

Banting, Frederick, 10, 12
Best, Charles, 10, 12
biguanides, 88–89
birth control, 127, 136
blindness, 61
brittle diabetes, 17, 111
bronchitis, 119
bulimia, 128

C

Cantani, Arnoldo, 91
cataracts, 61

cocaine, 117
Collip, J. B., 12

D

dehydration, 13, 69, 129
depression, 26, 27–28, 39,
80, 128
diabetes
being prepared, 122–123,
146–153
changes to your health,
59–69
diagnosis, 9, 15, 16, 18–22,
23, 36, 38, 40, 43, 45,
46, 49, 66, 70, 151
future of, 140–145
maintaining your health,
70–90
in males vs. females,
124–127
myths and facts, 46, 48,
93, 146, 152–153
in teens, 27, 31–32, 35,
116–130, 146
through time, 8–17, 38,
59, 78, 91, 100
types of, 13–17
who gets it, 23–30
your school and, 49–58
Diabetes Control and
Complications Trial
(DCCT), 78, 79

ABOUT THE AUTHOR

Leslie Green learned a great deal about diabetes while writing this book. She lives in Little Rock, Arkansas, with her three children and a pet turtle.

PHOTO CREDITS

Cover, back cover p. 1 © www.istockphoto.com/Fertnig; pp. 4, 20 Custom Medical Stock Photo; p. 9 History of Medicine/NIH; p. 11 Fotosearch/Archive Photos/Getty Images; p. 15 Jupiter Images/ Comstock/Thinkstock; pp. 22, 46–47, 69, 104, 108 istockphoto/ Thinkstock; p. 24 Peter Dazeley/Photographer's Choice/Getty Images; pp. 28, 76, 89, 148–149 Shutterstock; p. 32 Patrick Lane/ Blend Images/Getty Images; p. 41 © David Young-Wolff/Photo Edit; p. 50 © Tony Freeman/Photo Edit; p. 53 Ron Levine/Riser/Getty Images; p. 60 © David H. Lewis/www.istockphoto.com; pp. 65, 132 Phillippe Garo/Photo Researchers; pp. 66, 155 Courtesy of Jan S. Hittelman, Ph.D.; p. 72 © Mark Hatfield/www.istockphoto. com; p. 92 Banana Stock/Thinkstock; p. 97 Jupiterimages/FoodPix/ Getty Images; p. 99 Thinkstock Images/Comstock Images/Getty Images; p. 110 Dr. P. Marazzi/Photo Researchers; p. 119 Arthur Glauberman/Photo Researchers; p. 126 Reggie Casagrande/ Photographer's Choice/Getty Images; p. 141 David Sherman/ NBAE via Getty Images; p. 144 Newscom.

Editor: Bethany Bryan; Photo Researcher: Marty Levick